Anesthesia Equipment
Simplified

Anesthesia Equipment Simplified

Gregory Rose, MD
Associate Professor, Department of Anesthesiology
University of Kentucky College of Medicine
Lexington, Kentucky

J. Thomas McLarney, MD
Associate Professor, Department of Anesthesiology
University of Kentucky College of Medicine
Medical Director
Anesthesiology Preoperative Assessment Clinic
UK Healthcare
Lexington, Kentucky

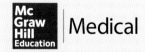

Medical

New York   Chicago   San Francisco   Athens   London   Madrid   Mexico City
Milan   New Delhi   Singapore   Sydney   Toronto

Anesthesia Equipment Simplified

1 2 3 4 5 6 7 8 9 0   CTP/CTP   18 17 16 15 14 13

ISBN 978-0-07-180518-6
MHID 0-07-180518-4

This book was set in Times New Roman PS by Thomson Digital.
The editors were Brian Belval and Christina M. Thomas.
The production supervisor was Catherine H. Saggese.
Project management was provided by Shaminder Pal Singh, Thomson Digital.
The cover designer was Thomas De Pierro.
China Translation & Printing Services, Ltd. was printer and binder.

This book is printed on acid-free paper.

Library of Congress Cataloging-in-Publication Data

Rose, Gregory (Gregory L.)
   Anesthesia equipment simplified / Gregory Rose, J. Thomas McLarney.
     p. ; cm.
   Includes bibliographical references and index.
   ISBN-13: 978-0-07-180518-6 (book : alk. paper)
   ISBN-10: 0-07-180518-4 (book : alk. paper)
   ISBN-13: 978-0-07-180519-3 (ebook)
   I. McLarney, J. Thomas. II. Title.
   [DNLM: 1. Anesthesiology—instrumentation. 2. Anesthetics, Inhalation.
3. Equipment Safety. 4. Ventilators, Mechanical—standards. WO 240]
   RD81
   617.9'6—dc23
                                                        2013010849

McGraw-Hill Education books are available at special quantity discounts to use as premiums and sales promotions, or for use in corporate training programs. To contact a representative please visit the Contact Us pages at www.mhprofessional.com.

This book is dedicated to all the resident physicians and students present and future who we hope will benefit from this work.

Contents

Preface

Anesthesia Equipment Simplified is the result of an idea that came to us during a discussion on how resident anesthesiologists have had such a hard time understanding how anesthesia equipment works, or not even acknowledging that the things we use every day of our clinical career are anything more than "black boxes" that are not meant to be understood by those who rely on them.

This is partially understandable, since there is such a myriad of knowledge and skill to obtain during one's residency. The resident physician anesthesiologist or student nurse anesthetist is busy studying subjects more related to life science and medicine in general. Physiology, anatomy, and pharmacology, the triad upon which our specialty is based, are things that we have at least some comfort level from our previous years of study; there are no classes in medical school on engineering.

It is in this light that we wrote *Anesthesia Equipment Simplified*: to make the understanding of the tools of our trades simpler for resident physicians, student nurse anesthetists, medical students, or anyone else who wants to really learn how these devices work.

Gregory Rose
J. Thomas McLarney

Acknowledgments

We are happy to be able to acknowledge those to whom we are indebted in the writing of this book. First and foremost we want to thank our Lord and Savior Jesus Christ for all his blessings that he has given us through the years. We wish to thank our chairman at the University of Kentucky College of Medicine, Dr. Edwin Bowe, for fostering and nurturing an environment in our anesthesiology department that allows for academic pursuits. We thank our colleague Dr. Eugene Hessel for his wonderful lectures during our training that sparked our interest in anesthesia equipment, and for reinforcing over the years the importance of knowing your equipment. Besides Dr. Bowe and Dr. Hessel, we are fortunate to have as a colleague Dr. John Eichhorn, whose name will be familiar to most as one of the leading experts on medical safety of his generation. He has answered many questions patiently for us through the years, and has helped us in our academic pursuits. Likewise, Dr. Raeford Brown of our department has been our mentor in our academic pursuits, and has been an enthusiastic supporter of our efforts in this project.

We also thank Dr. Thomas Murphy and Mr. Joseph Lesser, CRNA, members of our departmental equipment committee, for their work in evaluation of new equipment for our department, and for sharing their knowledge with us. Mr. Arthur Eversole is the biomedical technician in our operating rooms and has been a tremendous source of technical information for us over the years. Mr. Charles York has been exceptionally and cheerfully helpful as our staff assistant.

Brian Belval at McGraw-Hill has demonstrated the patience of Job during the production of this work, and we are grateful to him for expressing interest in this project. Christina Thomas of McGraw-Hill kept us on track for deadlines, and we are also grateful to her for her efforts. Sylvia Rebert, project manager, made the editing portion of this endeavor (which is new to us) painless and simple.

Finally, we wish to thank our families; Karen and Chris, and Tracy, Brannon, and Keegan, for bearing with us while we missed too many family dinners, too many soccer games, too many homework sessions, and too much yard work over the years during our medical practice and academic pursuits.

INTRODUCTION 1

Whether you are a practicing anesthesiologist, practicing nurse anesthetist, anesthesiology resident physician, or student nurse anesthetist, the chances are you know more about anatomy, pharmacology, and physiology than how the equipment that allows you to safely and properly give an anesthetic works. A lot of us are medically or biologically minded, not mechanically or electrically minded. That's one reason why we went into what we did instead of engineering. The workings of an anesthesia machine are not as interesting to us as the anatomy of a nerve block, how a drug works, or cardiac physiology.

The fact that anesthesia equipment isn't as interesting to us as the other things mentioned is understandable, but it is also dangerous. We, like some other medical personnel, must be able to quickly and correctly diagnose patient problems, but we must also be able to quickly and correctly diagnose what is wrong with our equipment. No specialty is as tied to its equipment as anesthesia. Of course, radiologists couldn't do much without x-ray machines, but they are usually not the ones who operate the machines, and besides, a patient won't die if the x-ray machine stops. But if our anesthesia machine stops working correctly, the patient can suffer harm. Therefore, we should know as much as possible about how our machines and equipment work so we can troubleshoot them effectively when necessary.

One of the physicians who we trained under said that we would check out the anesthesia machine much more carefully in the morning if our lives (and not just the life of the patient) depended on it, much like an airline pilot's life (and not just the lives of the passengers) depends on the proper functioning of his or her airplane. That is a true statement.

One of the things we have heard from the anesthesiology residents that we have trained over the years is that learning about anesthesia equipment is too difficult for someone who is not mechanically minded. The sources that exist to learn about how the tools of our trade work were impenetrable for some, so they simply ignored learning about anesthesia equipment. The goal of this book is stated in its title: to simplify the understanding of anesthesia equipment. That is not to say that we are not as serious about the subject as others;

our goal with this book is to provide simple, basic information on how all the wonderful equipment that we and our patients depend on actually works.

The chapters of this book are arranged in such a way as to follow the path that medical gases take through the anesthesia machine, starting with sources of medical gases and ending at the scavenger system. After that we discuss other anesthesia equipment that you use every day, but you might not know *how* the equipment actually works to assist you in providing a safe anesthetic. It is our sincere hope that *Anesthesia Equipment Simplified* lives up to its title in your mind.

OVERVIEW OF ANESTHESIA EQUIPMENT | 2

KEYWORDS

- design and ergonomics of anesthesia machines
- ASA monitoring standards

In this book, we will discuss different types of anesthesia equipment. When we say "anesthesia equipment," we mean the anesthesia machine itself, as well as the major monitoring devices. The trend is currently to have both machine and monitors integrated in an "anesthesia delivery system" or "anesthesia work station." Regardless of how the equipment is packaged, it is still useful to think of the components as separate entities in order to understand them. So in this book, when we talk about the "anesthesia machine," we mean the device that delivers oxygen and other gases, delivers inhalational anesthetics, and ventilates the patient. When we talk about "monitors," we generally mean the devices that measure physiologic, chemical, and pharmacologic information.

We will begin by reviewing what is found on a generic, modern anesthesia machine. It will be analogous to talking about airplanes; all airplanes fly, but there is a wide variety of designs, incorporating different engines, wings, and so forth, but all airplanes have things such as engines and wings. This is also how it is for anesthesia machines. They all do the same thing, but there are differences in how the same thing is done and differences in how machines are designed and function.

PURPOSE OF AN ANESTHESIA MACHINE

What is the main purpose of an anesthesia machine? This is a question we often ask medical students doing an anesthesia rotation. Naturally, many of them say something like "to deliver anesthesia gas to a patient." In our minds, that ability is not the main purpose of an anesthesia machine.

The main purpose of an anesthesia machine is to *deliver oxygen to a patient*. See the list below. Everything else is secondary. Everything about an anesthesia machine is built around the purpose of delivering oxygen to a patient. All the fail-safe systems of a machine concern the prevention of the delivery of a hypoxic mixture, not the delivery of anesthetic agents.

Okay, so what is the second most important function of an anesthesia machine? The students will then answer "to deliver anesthesia gas to a patient." But again they are wrong. After oxygenation, the next most important function or purpose of an anesthesia machine is to *provide a means of positive-pressure ventilation.* If we must ensure the patient receives oxygen, we must also have a means of being able to force oxygen into a patient because apnea is a major effect of anesthetics. Merely delivering oxygen to an apneic patient's mouth will not help too much.

Okay, so now comes the anesthesia delivery part, right? Yes, the third main function of an anesthesia machine is to *deliver inhalational anesthetic agents to a patient*. You should remember these functions in their order of importance as we go along.

MAIN PURPOSES OF AN ANESTHESIA MACHINE

1. Oxygen delivery
2. Means of positive-pressure ventilation
3. Delivery of inhalational anesthetics

GENERIC ANESTHESIA MACHINE

Let's pretend we are at an imaginary anesthesia machine dealer. We walk around, looking at all the shiny new models, enjoying that "new anesthesia machine smell," looking under the hoods, and so forth. They all may look different and have different options, but what kinds of things will we find on *every* one we look at?

Gases

There will be the capability to deliver at least two gases on an anesthesia machine: oxygen and nitrous oxide. Virtually all machines will also have medical air. (What about sevoflurane, desflurane, and isoflurane? Those things are *not* gases; more on this later on.)

When we say there is the capability to deliver specific gases, there will also be means of supplying the gases to the machine and controlling the flow rate and concentration of these gases.

Sources of Gases

A generic anesthesia machine will have the ability to obtain the gases from two different sources. One is from a gas pipeline, or "wall source." The other source is from medical gas cylinders. There will be built-in safety devices that will keep us from accidentally hooking a gas up to the wrong inlet of the machine so we will not inadvertently be delivering nitrous oxide when we think we are delivering oxygen. Additionally, there will be gauges, either electronic or analog, to tell us the pressure in psig (pounds per square inch) on the gauge of each source of each gas.

Flowmeters

Either electronic or glass flowmeters for each gas will be present, with control knobs for us to regulate both the concentration of gases and the flow rate in liters per minute.

Hypoxia Fail-Safe Devices

There are several different mechanisms that are built in to anesthesia machines that keep us from giving a hypoxic mixture of gases.

Vaporizers

After all, it *is* an anesthesia machine. There has to be a way of delivering inhalational anesthetic agents to the patient in a controllable, safe, efficient manner.

Reservoir Bag

This is the "squeeze bag" that we use to manually ventilate a patient. We must have a means of being able to deliver positive-pressure ventilation to the patient.

Ventilator

A means of automatically ventilating a patient is present on a generic anesthesia machine.

Circle Anesthesia Circuit

A circle circuit is by far the most commonly used anesthesia breathing circuit. This is the conduit from the machine to the patient that delivers oxygen and anesthetics and allows ventilation. There are several parts of a circle circuit as well, which are discussed in a later chapter.

Carbon Dioxide Absorber

A circle circuit means that there is rebreathing of carbon dioxide. Although it is true that there are types of anesthesia machines that are more like a critical care ventilator (semi-open circuit), virtually all anesthesia machines are semi-closed in function, meaning that there is rebreathing. So somehow we must be able to rid the rebreathed gas of carbon dioxide. A carbon dioxide absorber uses a chemical absorbent to scrub the rebreathed gas of carbon dioxide.

Waste Gas Scavenger

What happens to all of the inhalational agent that the patient is administered? It must go somewhere. It is true that there is rebreathing of the agent, but eventually it leaves the machine. A scavenger system allows the waste gas to leave the machine without polluting the working environment of the operating room (OR), sparing us from long-term exposure to the anesthetics.

Oxygen Flush System

For a multitude of reasons, at some time the clinician needs to fill the machine quickly with oxygen or increase the pressure inside the machine. An oxygen flush button allows that to happen.

Auxiliary Flowmeter

Not every anesthetic is a general anesthetic. We often administer oxygen via nasal cannula during neuraxial anesthetics or monitored anesthesia care (MAC). An extra oxygen flowmeter allows us to do so easily.

Battery Backup

Does your machine have a battery? If so, when was it last tested? Again, most modern anesthesia machines will have some sort of electrical backup supply.

Electrical Equipment

The anesthesia machine is an electrical machine. It has wires and cords, and somewhere it will have at least one circuit breaker. There will be power outlets on the back of the machine for plugging in accessory equipment and monitors. Many will have USB and Ethernet interfaces for use with an automated record system, for example.

Components of a Generic Anesthesia Machine

Gases

1. Sources of gases	8. Carbon dioxide absorber
2. Flowmeters	9. Waste gas scavenger system
3. Hypoxia fail-safe devices	10. Oxygen flush system
4. Vaporizers	11. Auxiliary flowmeter
5. Reservoir bag	12. Battery backup
6. Ventilator	13. Electrical equipment
7. Circle circuit	

ATYPICAL ANESTHESIA MACHINES

Not every anesthesia machine has everything on it. There are portable machines that can fit in a suitcase-sized container for use in office-based anesthesia. Such a machine might have room for only one vaporizer and might not have a ventilator incorporated into the unit itself. Still, a portable machine is capable of delivering inhalational anesthetics, albeit with less of a choice of agent selection, and still be able to give positive-pressure ventilation to a patient through a circle circuit. Another place where portable machines find use is in the military.

As mentioned, some anesthesia machines have a semi-open circuit, where there is no rebreathing and no need for a carbon dioxide absorber. These types of machines are modifications of critical care ventilators, with special vaporizers attached to deliver inhalational agent. The use of these machines was more common in the past, when the average OR anesthesia machine did not have enough driving force to properly ventilate a patient with stiff lungs. However, now the average anesthesia machine is much more able to adequately ventilate a patient with poor compliance.

MANUFACTURERS OF ANESTHESIA MACHINES

There are several manufacturers of anesthesia machines. It is safe to say, however, that the two biggest names in anesthesia machines are Draeger (North American Draeger) and General Electric. Draeger has been making anesthesia machines under the Draeger brand name for decades. General Electric (GE) is the other main manufacturer of anesthesia machines. The division of GE that makes anesthesia machines used to be called Datex Ohmeda (a brand name still used for anesthesia monitoring), so many machines in current use will still have the Datex Ohmeda brand name on them, and many clinicians will still call the GE models Ohmedas because of the history and common historical design features.

In some ways, this is all like automobile manufacturers; some people have a loyalty to Chevrolet and others to Ford, Chrysler, Toyota, or Mercedes. Many of us can tell the make of car we see by its appearance, and with a trained eye, many of us can tell the brand of machine by its appearance.

Another way anesthesia machines are comparable to automobiles is that whatever auto you buy, it will get you where you want to go. The same is true of anesthesia machines. Sometimes the choice of what machine a group will buy comes down to what company will give the group the better deal. Sometimes the buying group may desire certain features on one brand of anesthesia machine that are not on another. Other considerations include maintenance support, ease of servicing, brand loyalty, and so forth.

One final way that anesthesia machines are similar to automobiles is that the manufacturers give each model a name that might not have anything to do with its purpose. For instance, Draeger has a model called Apollo. It's a cool name but doesn't have much to do with anesthesia. GE has a model called Avance, which is a made-up name. Others use letters and numbers, such as the Maquet Flow –i C20.

Below is a list of anesthesia machine manufacturers in North America. The list is not inclusive but has most of the major companies.

Draeger
General Electric
Maquet
Spacelabs
Oceanic Medical
Cardinal Medical
Mindray
Braun

ANESTHESIA MONITORING

As anesthesia care providers, we are literally surrounded by monitors. It is possible to divide anesthesia monitoring devices into two groups: those that monitor *the patient* and those that monitor *the anesthetic.* What do we mean by that?

Patient Monitoring

Patient (or physiologic) monitoring means all the things we think of when we think of anesthesia monitoring—blood pressure, electrocardiography, heart rate, oxygen saturation, and so forth. These are things in which we find ourselves engrossed during a procedure. There are specific things that we must monitor during an anesthetic, and two of the first things we learn in training are *what* to monitor and *how* to monitor.

What to monitor and *how* to monitor are part of what makes up what is called *the standard of care*. Some things must be monitored, and failure to do so deviates from the standard of care (i.e., the level of care a patient undergoing an anesthetic should be given). In this book, we will discuss how monitors work, not how to interpret the information gathered.

There are many manufacturers of anesthesia physiologic monitoring equipment, more than we care to list. As we mentioned earlier, some monitors are incorporated into the anesthesia machine itself. In such cases, the company that makes the monitors is the same company that makes the machine. Other companies specialize in certain types of physiologic monitors. We will discuss physiologic monitoring in much more detail in other chapters.

Safety Monitoring

We have talked a little about the monitors we use to monitor the patient and mentioned that there are other monitors that monitor the anesthetic. We will explain what we mean.

Let's take blood pressure monitoring as an example of a means of monitoring the patient. In measuring blood pressure, we have a concrete, physiologically meaningful value, and as anesthesia personnel, we are able to evaluate and pharmacologically modify it if needed. The value has nothing to do with our equipment itself. It is like saying that an airliner is flying at 20,000 feet; knowing that fact does not tell the pilot that he or she is about ready to run out of fuel or hit a mountain or that one of the engines is overheating. For that kind of information, the pilot relies on *safety monitors*.

It's the same thing for us. We have monitors that tell us about our flight (patient) and those that tell us about our airplane (anesthesia machine). If you think of monitors in this way, you will appreciate the importance of the monitors that ensure we deliver a safe anesthetic.

History of Safety Monitoring

We all know the practice of anesthesia began in the 1840s. (If you didn't know that, you should. It's a fascinating story of many different people, of success and failure, of glory and even suicide. You owe it to your specialty to know its history.) The concept of safety monitoring did not come into widespread thought until the 1970s at the earliest, and it was not implemented until the mid 1980s!

The 1980s were an important time in anesthesia. Patient safety became a big concern. Some big names in our specialty began to discuss publically if a blood pressure cuff and a precordial stethoscope were adequate to give a safe anesthetic. In hindsight, we are astonished and would never think of anesthetizing anyone without our tremendous monitoring capability. Plenty of good clinicians thought that anesthesia was safe enough doing it *the same way* that it had been done for decades. Sure, there were bad outcomes, but they were few and far between. Some wondered, though, if adverse events could be made fewer and farther between.

The Anesthesia Patient Safety Foundation (APSF) was founded in 1985 by the then-president of the American Society of Anesthesiologists, E.C. "Jeep" Pierce, and others, including Robert Stoelting. It was their goal to create a "culture of safety" in the practice of anesthesia, and through the efforts of the APSF and their quarterly newsletter, they have succeeded. Anesthesiology has been one of the prime movers in advocating patient safety since.

One of the men most responsible for the concept of not only monitoring the patient but also monitoring the anesthetic is John Eichhorn. He was one of the co-authors of the "Harvard Standards," published in 1986 in the *Journal of the American Medical Association* (*JAMA*). The same standards, with minimal change, were adopted by the American Society of Anesthesiologists (ASA) as a *standard of care* soon after[1]. We are privileged to have him as a colleague in our department.

Monitoring Standards

Here is an abridged version of the 1986 ASA "Standards for Basic Intra-operative Monitoring."

Standard 1: Qualified anesthesia personnel shall be present in the room throughout the conduct of all general anesthetics, regional anesthetics, and monitored anesthesia care.

Standard 2: During all anesthetics, the patient's oxygenation, ventilation, circulation, and temperature shall be continually evaluated.

1. Inspired gas: During every administration of general anesthesia using an anesthesia machine, the concentration of oxygen in the patient breathing system shall be measured by an oxygen analyzer with a low oxygen concentration limit alarm in use.

2. Ventilation:

   A. Every patient receiving general anesthesia shall have the adequacy of ventilation continually evaluated. While qualitative clinical signs such as chest excursion, observation of the reservoir breathing bag, and auscultation of breath sounds may be adequate, quantitative monitoring of the CO_2 content and/or volume of expired gas is encouraged.

B. When an endotracheal tube is inserted, its correct positioning in the trachea must be verified. Clinical assessment is essential, and end-tidal CO_2 analysis, in use from the time of endotracheal tube placement, is encouraged.

C. When ventilation is controlled by a mechanical ventilator, there shall be in continuous use a device that is capable of detecting disconnection of components of the breathing system. The device must give an audible signal when its alarm threshold is exceeded.

D. During regional anesthesia and monitored anesthesia the adequacy of ventilation shall be evaluated, at least, by continual observation of qualitative clinical signs.

3. Circulation:

A. Every patient receiving anesthesia shall have the electrocardiogram continuously displayed from the beginning of anesthesia until preparing to leave the anesthetizing location.

B. Every patient receiving anesthesia shall have arterial blood pressure and heart rate determined and evaluated at least every five minutes.

C. Every patient receiving general anesthesia shall have, in addition to the above, circulatory function continually evaluated by at least one of the following; palpation of a pulse, auscultation of heart sounds, monitoring of a tracing of intra-arterial pressure, ultrasound peripheral pulse monitoring, or pulse plethysmography or oximetry.

4. Body Temperature:

A. Them shall be readily available a means to continuously monitor the patient's temperature When changes in body temperature are intended, anticipated or suspended, the temperature shall be measured. (Based on the ASA Standards for "Basic Intra-operative Monitoring" of the American Society of Anesthesiologists.)

We include these guidelines from 1986 to show you how different the practice of anesthesia used to be. You undoubtedly know anesthesia providers who practiced anesthesia before these standards actually *became* standards. Today none of us, including the more experienced of us who actually were giving anesthetics in 1986, would be comfortable anesthetizing anyone without the monitoring that these guidelines mandate. If you read close enough, you will see that even capnography was "encouraged," and pulse oximetry was only one of the accepted modalities of circulation monitoring. Today these are all things that we take for granted, and most of us have never given an anesthetic without the monitors mentioned above.

We believe that the mid 1980s was when the modern era of anesthesia began. The difference between this modern era and before was not the drugs given or the techniques used but the monitoring indicated, specifically monitoring that related to *safety*. An oxygen sensor is a *safety monitor*. Although capnography and pulse oximetry are used for physiologic monitoring, they are also *safety monitors*.

CONCLUSION

We do not want you to think that the practice of anesthesia before the 1980s was the dark ages, but the works of the individuals in the 1980s who created the culture of safety in anesthesia were responsible for decreasing the incidence of death for a healthy individual undergoing anesthesia from two to three per 10,000 to one per 100,000, which is about the chance of being struck by lightning. We have much to thank these people for. Their legacy of safety is enacted every time you calibrate your oxygen sensor or attach a pulse oximeter probe.

REFERENCE

1. Eichhorn JH. ASA adopts basic monitoring standards. *Anesthesia Patient Safety Foundation Newsletter* 1987;2(1):1–8.

MEDICAL GAS SUPPLY SYSTEMS | 3

There are many things that are a part of our lives, both personal and professional, that we take for granted. When we turn on the faucet, we expect water to come out; when we turn on the TV, we expect there is electricity flowing through the wires in the room so the TV comes on; and when we turn on an oxygen flowmeter, we expect oxygen to be there as well. But *how* does the medical facility in which you train or practice ensure that there is oxygen available when you turn on the flowmeter? Many of us might understand how we get the water to the tap or the electricity to the outlet better than we understand where the oxygen we use in great quantities every day comes from.

As a clinician, you will use much more oxygen in a day than you use water—did you ever think of that? So, it is a good idea to talk about where the medical gases we use get to the outlet for us and what would happen and what *you* would do if that supply was interrupted. Don't assume that somebody else will know what to do. It's *your* responsibility.

When we discuss medical gases, the big one is, of course, oxygen. We have the ability on our anesthesia machines to use oxygen from two different sources—cylinders and the hospital pipeline (wall) source. But you should remember that unless you always use cylinders of nitrous oxide and medical air, these two gases for your anesthesia machine come from the hospital supply as well.

In this chapter, we will discuss the systems that facilities use to supply oxygen, nitrous, and air via pipelines as well as some potential problems that can happen. We will also talk about how medical suction is generated and distributed throughout a building.

OXYGEN

Oxygen supplied through a medical pipeline system can have two sources: it can originate from a collection of large cylinders, or it can come from a liquid oxygen storage system. Smaller facilities, such as an outpatient surgery center that is not a part of a larger health care campus, will likely have a group of large oxygen cylinders as the source of pipeline oxygen. Hospitals, which will use thousands of liters of oxygen a day, use bulk liquid oxygen to supply their needs. We will discuss both kinds of sources.

Cylinder

In this setup, a group of "H" cylinders of oxygen will be attached to each other through a common manifold. The number of cylinders involved depends on the oxygen consumption of the facility—there can be as few as two or as many as the facility needs. There is a one-way valve between each tank and the common manifold, so if a tank has a leak or is empty, there will be no retrograde flow. From the manifold, the oxygen goes to a pressure regulator to take the pressure down to 50 to 55 psig, which is what pressure the oxygen is when it comes out of the wall pipeline. This setup is the *primary* supply. Some places also have a *secondary* supply as a backup.

The location of such a supply can be a small closet-sized area, a supply room, or an outdoor pen. It needs to be accessible to medical gas company workers for the cylinders to be changed out. Remember that an "H" cylinder holds 6900 L of oxygen at a pressure (when full) of 2200 psig, the same pressure as a full "E" cylinder. For a small hospital or surgery center, five to 10 "H" cylinders can supply several days' worth of oxygen. If a facility had five "H" tanks, that would be:

$$5 \text{ tanks} \times 6900 \text{ L} = 34{,}000 \text{ L}$$

So if a surgery center had five rooms, and we say the average oxygen use per anesthesia machine is 3 L/min:

$$5 \text{ machines} \times 3 \text{ L/min} \times 60 \text{ minutes} = 900 \text{ L/hr}$$

And then

$$900 \text{ L/hr} \times 8 \text{ hr} = 7{,}200 \text{ L/day}$$

So

$$34{,}000 \text{ L} \div 7200 \text{ L/day} = 4.7 \text{ days' worth of oxygen}$$

Are you comfortable with that supply of oxygen? A facility has to figure in how much the delivery costs are for the gas distributor to come out every

4 days. More cylinders might be better. Also keep in mind that oxygen consumption goes on not only in the operating room (OR) but also in the recovery room, intensive care units, or anywhere procedures are done such as the cath lab, endoscopy, and interventional radiology.

This is also a good place to discuss actual oxygen use of your anesthesia machine. Does anything else on your anesthesia machine use oxygen besides what you dial in with your flowmeter? This is an example of why it is important to know as much about the anesthesia machine as you can. As discussed in the chapter on anesthesia ventilators, the type of anesthesia machine you use makes an incredible difference in oxygen usage. A piston ventilator uses no oxygen other than what is dialed into the flowmeter. A Datex-Ohmeda bellows ventilator uses a quantity of oxygen more or less equal to the patient's minute ventilation in addition to what is going through the flowmeter (a Draeger bellows ventilator uses a mixture of oxygen and air, but Draeger no longer makes bellows ventilators). If oxygen supply is a consideration, you might want to consider piston drive ventilators the next time the facility purchases new machines.

Liquid Oxygen

This is the manner in which most large hospitals store oxygen. It is more economical than using dozens of cylinders a day. Liquid oxygen is powerful stuff; it is used in rocket propulsion. Fortunately, it has been learned over the years how to handle and store it relatively safely.

Somewhere outside around your hospital there will be at least one big white tank. This is the liquid oxygen storage tank. It must be accessible to the traffic of large tractor-trailer–sized vehicles that come periodically to refill it. The tank itself is like a Thermos bottle. It has an inner lining, a space for insulation, and an outer shell. Remember that liquid oxygen is *very* cold. It is moved and stored at a temperature of somewhere below its boiling point, which is −297°F.

Even with the insulated tank, some of the liquid oxygen will go from liquid to gas because of the loss of cold from the outside environment. So at any time in the tank there will be some gaseous oxygen and some liquid oxygen. To keep the pressure from getting too high in the tank, relief valves are present to vent off the gaseous oxygen if the internal pressure reaches a certain point. A whole system of pressure sensors and volume measurements makes sure the system is functioning properly and lets people know when it is time to refill the tank. A smaller backup tank is present in many situations to be used when the main tank undergoes maintenance or experiences a problem.

Of course, the oxygen that comes out of our pipeline source is not anywhere near −297°F. How does the oxygen warm up? With usage, liquid oxygen is drawn out of the tank and goes through a vaporizer. It is not the same type of vaporizer that we have to administer anesthetic agents with on our anesthesia machines. This kind of vaporizer is a warming system for the oxygen. Using hot water or other type of electrically generated heat, the liquid oxygen is changed into gas. Then it goes into the hospital pipeline system.

This kind of system works very well, and there are people at your hospital whose job is to make sure everything goes okay with all this equipment. But what kind of things can go wrong?

Because there are a lot of pipes and connections, leaks can occur. Valves can malfunction, causing release of too much oxygen and depleting supply. Selector switches can malfunction, causing the backup supply to be used instead of the main source. Pipes and tubing can burst. A large vehicle can back into the main tank, causing catastrophic loss of oxygen supply.

In 2004 at the University of Alabama Medical Center in Birmingham, a catastrophic oxygen tank malfunction occurred. A large pipe connection failed, and 8000 gallons of liquid oxygen escaped, covering the immediate area around the tank with a dense, cold fog. The engineers had trouble checking the function of the backup system because it was close enough to the large tank that the conditions obscured the backup tank. The hospital staff quickly changed over to oxygen cylinders as their source and began oxygen-conserving measures. The engineering department was able to put online another interconnected bulk oxygen source from a block away.

So as you see, things *really can* go wrong with oxygen supply. We hope any future events such as this will be handled as well as it was in this circumstance.

Oxygen Concentrators

These units are mainly for individual use, but steps to make large systems appropriate for generating amounts needed for institutional use are underway. Concentrators rely on a substance called zeolite, which is a family of aluminosilicate minerals. Zeolites absorb things and are used in things ranging from water purification to cat litter. Zeolite absorbs nitrogen when pressurized ambient air is forced through a canister of it, leaving oxygen and the other things found in regular air such as water vapor and argon. The zeolite becomes saturated quickly, so after a few seconds, the air compressor in the unit switches to a different zeolite canister, and the first canister of zeolite quickly releases its nitrogen. The zeolite is reusable in this manner over and over and over again.

NITROUS OXIDE

Nitrous oxide is stored in bulk supply at facilities using multiple large cylinders all connected to a large manifold, as we discussed earlier with bulk oxygen cylinder storage.

MEDICAL AIR

Supplying air to the pipelines seems like it would be simple. A bunch of air tanks attached by a manifold would do the job, right? Actually, virtually all facilities produce their own medical air. It is cheaper in the long run than to get the supply from cylinders from a gas supplier.

So, can't we go to a "big box" store and buy an air compressor or even two or three to meet the possible demand? No, it is more complicated than that as well. Believe it or not, medical air is considered a drug. It has to undergo processing and filtering to ensure that it is appropriate for patient use and for use in various types of medical equipment.

Let's start at the beginning of the process of creating medical-grade air. This will take us to the roof of the facility in question. There are guidelines for where the intake should be. It needs to be 10 feet from any door or window or other duct or vent (similar to the exhaust line for hospital suction or the anesthesia scavenger system). It needs to be at least 20 feet above the ground (which, usually on the monstrous buildings in which we practice, is not a problem). It needs to be far enough away from sources of pollution, such as loading docks and helipads, so engine exhaust does not get into the source. The intake pipe is curved so that the opening faces downward, so precipitation and particulate matter do not fall into it. It must have a screen over the opening so birds will not fly into it or nest in it.

Before you think this is all much ado about nothing, there have been instances when medical gas lines were found to have dead animals in them, which caused a big stink in more than one way. Also, when hospitals have expanded or added a helipad, the "prevailing wind" of air on the roof was changed so that the exhaust from delivery trucks or the helicopter contaminated the medical air that was produced by the hospital. Allowing carbon monoxide exhaust into a patient's air supply is not a good thing. If there is enough local pollution that it is unfeasible to use outside air, it is proper to obtain air from *inside* the facility to process into medical air. If that is not feasible, medical air cylinders may have to be used.

There may be particle filters that are located between the intake and the compressors themselves. There will be at least two compressors (in case one stops working), but a big hospital will have more than that. These compressors are designed differently than the one you may have in your garage, so no oil from the machinery can get into the compressed air that is produced.

Compressing the air causes heat. So after the air leaves the compressor itself, it goes through a cooling system. This allows moisture in the warm air to rain out into water traps along the way because medical air needs to be very dry. A large tank stores the medical gas that is produced. If the tank gets too full, there is a relief valve to vent it, and a control system will shut down the compressors until more air is needed to keep the tank capacity at a proper level.

After leaving the storage tank, the gas will go through more filters to remove particulates. Again, these are not the same kind of filter in your home heating and air conditioning system. The filters must catch particles down to at least 1 micron at a flow rate of 100% of the system's capability. Small particles of oil, rust, pollen, spores, and so forth are filtered out of the system, and more water is removed at this stage.

When it comes out of the compression and filtration system, the air is at a higher pressure than what we want it to be for our use (50–55 psig), so pressure regulators decrease its pressure before it gets into the main hospital system.

By the way, hospital pipelines are made from metal such as copper or brass, not iron or steel, so they will not rust and fail over time. PVC pipe may be good enough at home for some uses but not for hospital gas systems.

Please remember this: if there is any construction going on in or around the OR or anywhere in the facility, remember that medical gas pipelines have been connected improperly before, and patients have died from getting nitrous oxide instead of oxygen. That is why oxygen measurement in the inspiratory limb of your anesthesia machine circuit is important.

MEDICAL SUCTION

Suction is something that we think even less about where it comes from than our pipeline gases. The only time we talk about suction is when something is wrong with it. "Who took my suction?," "Can you check my suction please?," and "The suction's not working!" are cries that are commonly heard in ORs and often are the only time suction is mentioned. In a way, suction is similar to the practice of anesthesia: both are expected to always be flawless in performance but are often not considered until something goes wrong with either.

Medical suction is generated in sort of the opposite way of medical air: a vacuum pump is similar to an air compressor; the business end of one is pushing air out, and the other is sucking it in. Similar to the inlet for medical air, the outlet for suction is on the roof and at least 10 feet from the medical air inlet. In fact, the farther it is from the medical air inlet, the better it is. Think of all the stuff that would come out of a medical suction outlet—unpleasant odors, maybe pathogens, nitrous oxide, inhalational agents, and so on. The outlet pipe needs to be curved so the outlet itself faces downward and needs to have a screen on it to keep birds out.

Between the vacuum pump and the user interface will be a tank that functions like a large suction canister, catching liquids and solids that may have gotten into the pipeline during use. Also, a small bottle is often attached to the wall at the suction inlet to catch anything that escapes the suction canister. The disposable suction canisters may have a float valve that will occlude the suction canister if it gets too full to keep the contents from going into the wall. There is a vacuum regulator with a negative-pressure gauge between the canister and the user to regulate the power of suction required. In clinical practice, the regulator is set at full most of the time to ensure rapid suctioning of the airway when needed.

How strong does the suction need to be? The minimum requirement is that suction at the outlet farthest from the vacuum pump system needs to generate a negative pressure of at least 12 mm Hg.

There are other forms of suction available besides wall suction. In the past, smaller suction machines were common in ORs before hospital-wide suction systems became the norm. Known generically as "gomcos" after one of the top manufacturers (Goldstein Medical Company), they are still found in smaller health care settings such as offices, clinics, and even ambulances and medical helicopters. They can generate as much vacuum as the wall-source systems and have a canister system to hold the suctioned liquid. These units run on electricity, and some are equipped with batteries in case of a power loss. There are also portable units that rely on manual or foot pedal power to generate suction for field use.

At the business end of the suction system is a suction catheter. There are various kinds, as you know. Some are for suctioning endotracheal tubes. Some are combination cautery–suction devices for surgical procedures. There is a pool suction tip for draining large amounts of fluid. But the suction catheter most widely used is the Yankauer suction tip. But have you ever wondered who or what is a "Yankauer"?

Charles Yankauer was an ear, nose, and throat physician who, around the turn of the twentieth century, designed the suction tip that we use so much. He designed it with surgical use in mind, however—long but small in diameter to not hinder his view when working in the pharynx and with orifices of a size appropriate for blood and saliva to be suctioned effectively. It nevertheless was adopted long ago by anesthesiologists and anesthetists to be our main suction device. It is long enough for our purposes and small enough in caliber to squeeze into a patient's mouth on emergence. But if you have ever tried to suction stomach contents out of a pharynx with one, you wished it had a larger capacity in regards to not only volume but also particle size.

CONCLUSION

We are hopeful that now you have a better understanding of where your pipeline supply comes from and goes to as well as suction systems. You will also have a better appreciation of how much we rely on these systems and an appreciation for the people who keep them running.

PNEUMATIC SYSTEMS

KEYWORDS

- oxygen
- nitrous oxide
- medical air
- design of anesthesia machines
- oxygen supply systems
- medical gas cylinders
- regulators

In this chapter, we will discuss how our medical gases (oxygen, nitrous oxide, and air) get into the machine and what happens to them when they are in there. The pneumatic system of an anesthesia machine is subdivided into three smaller systems based on the amount of pressure seen in each one: the *high-pressure system* (concerning the gas cylinders on the back of the machine), the *intermediate-pressure system* (concerning gases from the pipeline or wall source), and the *low-pressure system* (flowmeters). We will discuss the first two in this chapter and will cover flowmeters in a separate chapter.

HIGH-PRESSURE SYSTEM

This system includes the gas cylinders, or tanks, on the back of the machine; how the cylinders are mounted onto the hanger yoke on the back of the machine; and what happens to the gas after it enters the machine.

Cylinders

Volumes and Pressure

We are all familiar with the "E" cylinders that are mounted on the backs of anesthesia machines and used for patient transport. An E cylinder of oxygen that is full contains 660 L of oxygen and is at a pressure of 2,200 psig. An E cylinder of nitrous oxide has 1590 L at a pressure of 745 psig.

An oxygen cylinder has a linear relationship between volume and pressure; for example, when the cylinder is half empty, at 330 L, the pressure will be around 1100 psig, and so on, until the tank is empty.

A nitrous oxide cylinder, when full, has some of its contents in a gaseous phase and some in a liquid phase. The pounds per square inch of a nitrous oxide cylinder will read 745 throughout most of its useful life. That is because there is a nonlinear relationship between volume and pressure in regards to nitrous oxide because part of it is in a liquid phase. As long as there is liquid in the tank contributing to the vapor pressure of the gas above it, the pressure gauge will not change.

That is why it is recommended to change nitrous oxide cylinders when the pressure begins to read below 745 psig. There can still be a good amount of nitrous oxide in the tank (up to 400 L) when the liquid nitrous oxide is gone, but there is no way of knowing except to take the tank off the back of the machine and weigh it. Even if you wanted to weigh the existing tank, when it is off the machine, it is easier in the long run to replace it with a full tank and not worry about how much nitrous oxide is left.

Cylinder Color

An oxygen cylinder is green, right? Have you ever seen one that is not green? Well, if you have been practicing anesthesia outside the United States, you have seen oxygen tanks of a different color. Medical gas colors can be different in different parts of the world. Although we rely on color very much in our specialty (gases, inhalational agents, oral airway sizes, and so on), color coding is *not* foolproof.

Did you know that it is not a law or a Food and Drug Administration regulation that oxygen is always in a green tank, nitrous oxide is always in a blue tank, or air is always in a yellow tank? It is a guideline but not a requirement. All that your local medical gas supplier needs to do to be legal is to properly *label* the tank for its contents. The authors once discovered an air tank attached to our machine that was gray, similar to a cylinder of carbon dioxide. Gas analysis proved the contents were in fact air, and the tank was labeled as medical air.

Correct Gas Placement

Now are you worried that you may put a gas cylinder onto a wrong yoke on the back of the machine? That is why it is important to *read* labels. Color coding is helpful, but we have seen that it can potentially mislead you.

Fortunately, there is another way to ensure placing the correct tank onto the correct yoke. On the stem of each gas cylinder (the stem is the chrome part on the very top of the cylinder) are a couple of little holes that line up with a couple of little pins right where the stem fits onto the yoke nipple. The pins and holes are in matching positions that are different for each gas. This

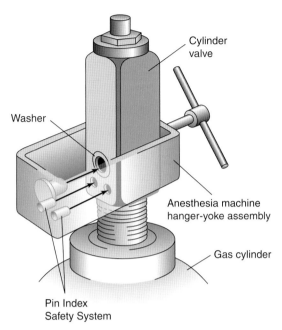

Cylinder valve

Washer

Anesthesia machine hanger-yoke assembly

Gas cylinder

Pin Index Safety System

Figure 4-1 ▪ Pin Index Safety System interlink between the anesthesia machine and gas cylinder. (Reproduced with permission from Morgan GE, Mikhail MS, Murray MJ. *Clinical Anesthesiology.* 4th ed. New York, NY: McGraw-Hill; 2006. Figure 2-4.)

is called the Pin Index Safety System (Figure 4-1). If the pins on the yoke do not line up with the holes on the cylinder stem of a corresponding tank, get another cylinder and check the yoke. Either the cylinder has an incorrect stem on it or the yoke pins have been damaged (Figure 4-2). To proceed with a case using that cylinder or yoke is not a good idea.

We all rely on anesthesia technicians and other ancillary staff to help us in our daily work. They may even know more about the machine than we do. But don't count on it. A pilot doesn't trust the baggage handler to check out the avionics of the plane, and we shouldn't rely solely on staff to know more about the machine than we do. While it is true a pilot probably doesn't know how to refuel his airliner, we *should* know how to replace a cylinder. If you don't, make it a priority to learn how.

A full cylinder should come with a new washer taped or somehow attached to the stem. This washer is what goes between the cylinder and the yoke nipple. If it is not placed there, there will be a leak when the cylinder is opened. The exit of pressurized gas from a cylinder to the machine inlet results in heat, which can deform and flatten the washer. That is why a new washer should be used each time a cylinder is changed.

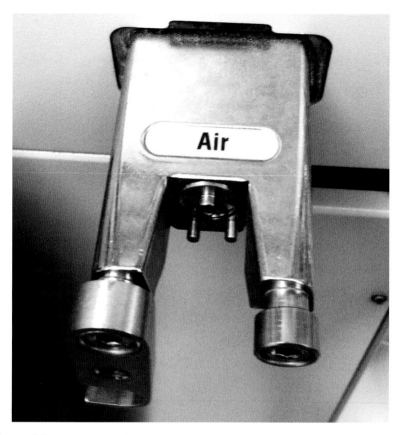

Figure 4-2 ▪ Empty air yoke showing Pin Index Safety System pins.

Be sure to take the old washer off, though! If more than one washer is used between the cylinder stem and the yoke nipple, the added space the extra washer creates can be enough to inadvertently disable the Pin Index Safety System by making the pins unable to reach the corresponding holes.

Check Valve

A machine should always have an oxygen cylinder on it. Some types of machines even have two yokes for oxygen. It is less important to have nitrous oxide and air cylinders on their yokes, of course, because they are not absolutely necessary to safely perform an anesthetic. So why isn't there a leak from empty yokes when you are using pipeline gas?

There is a check valve for each yoke. When the pressure of the gas in the cylinder is greater than that of the gas in the machine (meaning when you have opened the cylinder), the check valve is opened by that pressure. When

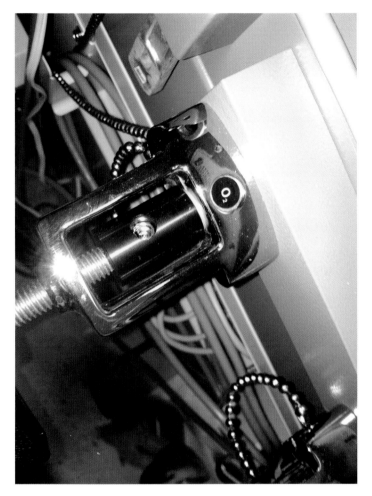

Figure 4-3 ▪ Draeger yoke plug.

the pressure in the machine is greater than the pressure of an empty cylinder or there is no cylinder on the yoke, the check valve closes. But even with this check valve system, a small amount of gas from inside the machine can escape from around the closed check valve if the yoke is empty. Gas-specific yoke plugs are available that stop these kind of small leaks (Figure 4-3).

Pressure Gauge

All anesthesia machines have a means of measuring the pressure of each cylinder attached to it. Some machines have traditional pressure gauges, which are round with the arrow pointing to the pressure level. Other machines have digital readouts of pressure (Figure 4-4).

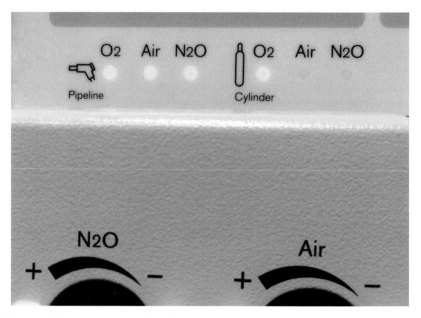

Figure 4-4 ▪ Draeger Apollo electronic gas pressure indicators, located above flowmeters, for both pipeline and cylinder sources. Actual pressure readouts on this machine are found on digital screen.

Pressure Regulator

The pressure in a full oxygen cylinder is 2200 psig. That is equal to 150 atmospheres! If you opened an oxygen cylinder and let 150 atmospheres travel through the machine, the machine wouldn't last long. The flowmeters would shatter, tubing would burst, and pieces would be flying off like an explosion inside the machine, which is more or less another way of describing the situation.

In addition, as gas leaves a cylinder, the cylinder pressure drops (except for nitrous oxide, which we discussed earlier; its pressure stays the same and then drops relatively suddenly as the tank is depleted). The regulator keeps the operator from having to adjust flow rates as the cylinder supply is used.

To make the pressure more manageable, there is a pressure regulator. It is also called a pressure reducing valve, regulator valve, and other variations of those words. How a pressure regulator works can be found in great detail in other texts. What you need to know is that the regulator is between the cylinders and the rest of the pneumatic system of the anesthesia machine. There is a pressure regulator not only for each gas but for each yoke. The pressure is reduced by the regulator from whatever the cylinder pressure is to 45 psig.

Why 45 psig? The pressure of the pipeline supply is 50 psig, so the regulator is designed to close itself when the pressure inside the machine (from the pipeline source) is greater than the regulator outlet pressure. That way, you don't use up your cylinder supply accidentally while you are attached to the pipeline, thereby keeping your tanks full for when you really need them.

It is important to keep your cylinders closed while you are using the pipeline source. There are a couple of reasons.

If your oxygen tank was open while you were using pipeline oxygen and if there was an actual loss of pipeline oxygen, the low oxygen alarm would not sound because there would be a relatively seamless transfer of delivery of oxygen from the now-dead pipeline supply to the left-open cylinder. Of course, the change would show up on the pressure gauges on the front of the machine, but realistically, how often do you look at the pressure gauges during a case? Therefore, the only time the low oxygen alarm would sound would be when the *cylinder is empty*.

So now you are blindsided by the fact that you have *no oxygen* at all. If the cylinder had been closed when the pipeline was lost, the alarm would have sounded, so you would have been alerted that there is a big problem with oxygen delivery. Then you could have simply opened your oxygen cylinder and made arrangements to get more full cylinders and changed your technique to save on oxygen use.

The other reason to keep your oxygen tank closed is in the case that the pipeline source pressure falls below 45 psig. Because of the preferential check valve between the high- and intermediate-pressure systems (which will close off the system with lower pressure), if your pipeline pressure falls below 45 psig, the check valve will close off the pipeline and begin using your cylinder oxygen, thereby wasting your backup oxygen source. Even if the pipeline pressure fell below 45 psig, there would still be enough oxygen to supply the machine and the patient.

Also along the way, from the tanks to the regulator, are filters to catch any particulate matter that may have found its way into the tanks at some point.

Is this confusing? We hope not. If so, read it again. Keep in mind that this whole system, the high-pressure system, deals *only* with the supply of gases coming from the cylinders on the back of your machine. Now to review:

- There is a way to safely ensure the correct gas cylinder is placed on the correct yoke on the back of the machine (Pin Index Safety System).
- There is a way to keep gas from leaking out of an empty yoke (check valve).
- There is a way to reduce the large pressure of the cylinders to a usable and safe pressure (pressure regulator).
- There is a way to know approximately how much gas you have in your cylinders and what the pressure is, and that cylinders are attached to your machine and are open (cylinder pressure gauges).

Table 4-1 **PARTS OF AN HIGH-PRESSURE PNEUMATIC SYSTEM**	
Gas cylinders	Gas machine yokes
Check valve	Pressure regulator
Cylinder pressure gauges	Filters

The parts of a high-pressure pneumatic system are summarized in Table 4-1.

Now we will begin discussing the system that deals with the pipeline source of gases—the intermediate-pressure system.

INTERMEDIATE–PRESSURE SYSTEM

This system deals with gases that come from two different places—the pressure regulators of the gas cylinders that we have just discussed and the wall pipeline source.

Pipeline Source

Anesthesia machines have two possible sources of the gases needed—the cylinders, or tanks on the back of the machine or the gas pipeline, or wall source of the facility. Most of the time, we use the pipeline supply because the machine is stationary whatever room it is in. We have a convenient source of gases, relatively unlimited compared with cylinders that we have to watch closely for when they become empty and have to be lugged around and switched out.

Cylinders are for when we must be in a location where there is no pipeline source, but mainly we have cylinders for the unlikely but extremely serious problem of losing our pipeline supply. Loss of pipeline supply is reported rarely but enough to get our attention. Pipes can break, a worker who doesn't know what he is doing can turn off the gas to your location, or a truck can back into the big white tank in back of the hospital and cause a spill of liquid oxygen that turns the oxygen tank into a huge fog machine. The bottom line is that *it can happen.* Loss of pipeline oxygen is similar to malignant hyperthermia: it may never happen to you in your career, but if it ever does, you need to recognize it immediately and know what to do.

So what do you do? Of course, you will open your oxygen cylinder on the back of the machine. The other important thing to do is to *disconnect* the oxygen hose from the pipeline outlet. Why? Remember from our earlier discussion about the pressure regulators that decrease the high pressure of the cylinders to 45 psig? Remember that we also said there is a check valve between the pipeline source and the cylinder source that opens for the higher pressure, which when things are okay will be the pipeline source (50 psig), to keep us from wasting our cylinder of oxygen when we are hooked up to the oxygen pipeline?

But if there is no oxygen coming out of the pipeline, what difference does it make if you don't disconnect the oxygen pipeline? When the oxygen pipeline source is finally fixed and is up and running, there may be particulate matter, grease, oil, or who knows what coming out of the pipeline initially. More disturbing is that pipelines may have been crossed in all the rush for the facility to reestablish pipeline oxygen. What could be coming out of the pipeline could be medical air, or worse, nitrous oxide.

The literature is full of reports of deaths from patients receiving nitrous oxide when the anesthetist thought oxygen was being administered. *It can happen.* Always be vigilant when construction is going on in or around the operating room because gas supply lines can be crossed. Always check what is coming out of the pipeline after renovations or new construction. The literature is full of reports of deaths at new facilities because no one had checked to see if oxygen was really coming out of the new oxygen pipeline.

Pipeline Connections

Similar to our discussion earlier about not putting a gas cylinder onto the wrong yoke on the back of a machine, how can we make sure we hook up the correct hoses to the correct pipeline outlets? Similar to cylinders, the gas hosing is color coded. The outlets are probably color coded also. But we saw that color coding has its drawbacks. We need a relatively foolproof system, such as the Pin Index Safety System.

Analogous to the Pin Index Safety System is the Diameter Index Safety System (Figure 4-5). The gas hosing has attachments on its distal end, varying in diameter and shape, that will only mate with its pipeline outlet counterpart. This system is also used for hospital suction and scavenging lines. In addition, the end that goes into the machine has threaded inlets that are of different diameters for the different gases, so an incorrect hose hookup cannot occur on that end, either. The inlets that are on the machine itself are actually the Diameter Index Safety System, not the ends of the hoses that go into the wall outlet. These ends that attach to the wall can vary in design from place to place. The pipeline hose inlets (where the hose attaches to the machine) each have a filter to catch particulate material. The inlets also have check valves to prevent loss of volume if the hoses are unused and not attached to the pipeline source (e.g., when you are running on cylinders or if you are not hooked up to nonessential nitrous oxide and air pipeline outlets).

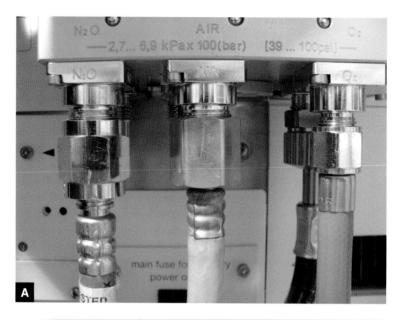

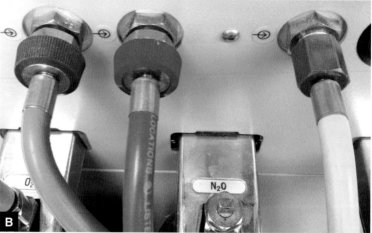

Figure 4-5 ■ Diameter Index Safety System of a Draeger machine (**A**) and a Datex-Ohmeda machine (**B**). The inlet for each gas is of a different diameter.

Pressure Gauge

Similar to the high-pressure system, the intermediate-pressure system has pressure measuring devices, either analog or digital, for the operator to check and watch. You should obviously be familiar with where on the machine you are using the readout is located. On newer machines, you may have to scroll through different pages on the information screen to find it.

Oxygen Flush

Every anesthesia machine has a large green button somewhere on the front of it. The button is recessed or has a guard around it so it will not be pushed accidentally. Pressing this button causes oxygen to come directly from the pipeline source (50 psig) or the cylinder pressure regulator (45 psig) and enter the low-pressure system downstream of the vaporizers at the common gas outlet. This is useful when you are having a difficult time with a facemask leak, to keep volume in your circuit. It is also useful at the end of a case to flush out your machine of agent to get your inspired agent concentration as low as possible or to rapidly decrease your inspired agent concentration if a patient is hypotensive. *But you must disconnect the circuit* from the patient before you use the flush button when flushing agent out of your machine. The high flow rates of oxygen (anywhere from 35 to 75 L/min) can cause barotrauma. Also, put your thumb over the end of the circuit so the room is not polluted with anesthetic agent.

Some models of anesthesia machines have oxygen flush systems that can be used as the source for jet ventilation. Some do not. An auxiliary oxygen flowmeter is better suited for jet ventilation anyway (Figure 4-6).

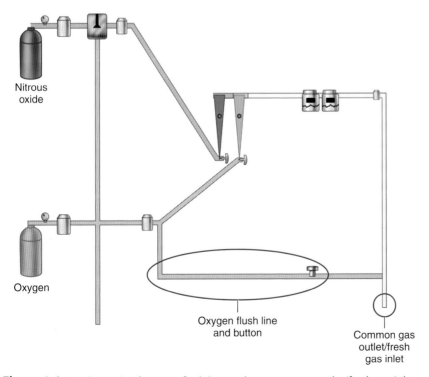

Nitrous oxide

Oxygen

Oxygen flush line and button

Common gas outlet/fresh gas inlet

Figure 4-6 ▪ Schematic of oxygen flush line and common gas outlet/fresh gas inlet.

Table 4-2 **PARTS OF AN INTERMEDIATE-PRESSURE PNEUMATIC SYSTEM**	
Gas pipeline sources	Input from high-pressure system
Pressure gauges	Oxygen flush
Secondary regulator (in some types)	

Undoubtedly the thing that the flush button is used the most for is to pressurize your circle circuit with your thumb over the Y-piece when you check your machine for leaks before each case.

Pressure Regulator

Yes, there is a pressure regulator for the intermediate-pressure system also but only in some models of anesthesia machines. The goal is to decrease pressure to around 26 psig so the flow from the pipeline is more even and smooth. The parts of an intermediate-pressure pneumatic system are summarized in Table 4-2.

There are additional things that are considered to be a part of the high- or intermediate-pressure systems, such as fail-safe devices and the pneumatic on/off control. These are presented in other chapters, and as mentioned earlier, we will discuss flowmeters (and what is called the low-pressure system) separately as well.

CONCLUSION

We hope that you have a better understanding of the pneumatic system of anesthesia machines and that you realize why it is important for you to understand how it functions.

FLOWMETERS AND THE LOW-PRESSURE SYSTEM

5

KEYWORDS

- flowmeters
- rotameter
- laminar-turbulent flow
- rotameter configuration

Similar to vaporizers, flowmeters are one of our interfaces with the anesthesia machine. Here is something that we can actually see in action. But there is more than meets the eye, as we will see. Flowmeters are part of the low-pressure system of the pneumatic part of the machine along with the high- and intermediate-pressure systems discussed in earlier chapters.

LOW-PRESSURE SYSTEM

Technically, the low-pressure system is everything that is downstream of the flow control valves. This includes the flowmeters themselves, vaporizers, and one-way valves (to decrease pumping; discussed in the vaporizer Chapter 6) and ends at the common gas outlet (which is the end of the pneumatic part of the machine and the beginning of the ventilator part of the machine).

FLOWMETERS AND THEIR PARTS

Flow Control Valve

The flow control valve is simply the thing attached to the knob we turn to adjust flow through the flowmeters. On most machines, flow control still uses a mechanical valve that is directly attached to one of the three knobs that are used to manipulate the flowmeters. However, some machines use electronic controls as the interface between the operator and the flowmeters.

With electronic flow control valves, the user may dial in the fraction of inspired oxygen (FiO_2) that is desired and which other gas to use to dilute the oxygen (nitrous oxide or air). The mixture is controlled by pressure sensors and may have input from the gas monitor or oxygen analyzer to maintain the concentration of oxygen that has been selected. The total fresh gas flow (FGF) with electronic flow control valves is set by yet another controller, instead of the standard way of controlling FGF via flow control valves with flowmeters. Electronic flow control valves thus allow a very exact control of oxygen concentration but with the penalty of needing electrical or battery power, something that traditional flow control valves and flowmeters do not need to function.

Control Knobs

You have probably noticed that the control knobs for the three different gases are color coded. The oxygen button and flowmeter are always on the right (more on that later). In addition, the oxygen knob is bigger and juts out more than the other two knobs. It is also fluted, so it feels different. That is all, of course, so when you need to increase the oxygen flow, you will with time know which one to change simply by touch and feel and not have to divert your eyes from the patient or monitors; you will instinctively know the most important of the three knobs by touch and not inadvertently change the air or nitrous oxide. All three of the knobs have some sort of guard around them to decrease the chance of the knobs being accidentally adjusted if something bumps into them. On standard flowmeters, turning the knob counterclockwise increases gas flow, and turning the knob clockwise decreases flow.

Machines with electronic flow control interfaces will not have the kind of knobs just described. Instead, they have touchpads to indicate which gas you want to change and a common knob that is used to change flow in whatever gas you have pushed the button for (Figure 5-1).

Flowmeter

Although most of us would think of the flowmeter as the control knob and the glass tubing; to be specific, the flowmeter is actually the part that is controlled by the knob, where we see the bobbin going up and down. Another name for a flowmeter is a *rotameter*.

You can go into the physics of flowmeters as deeply as you want. For our discussion, we will not delve too deeply. A flowmeter tube of the standard type is called a Thorpe tube. This kind of tube is made out of glass to keep a static electricity charge from building up on the bobbin inside and causing

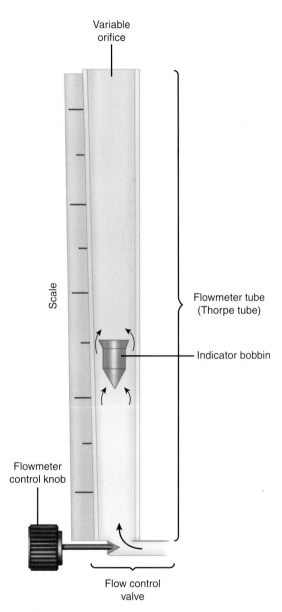

Figure 5-1 ▪ Simple schematic of a flowmeter with labeling. (Reproduced with permission from Morgan GE, Mikhail MS, Murray MJ. *Clinical Anesthesiology*. 2nd ed. New York, NY: McGraw-Hill; 2002. Figure 4-4.)

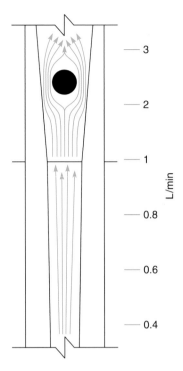

Figure 5-2 ▪ Illustration of an annular ring, the air space surrounding the bobbin or ball (*blue arrows*). (Reproduced with permission from Morgan GE, Mikhail MS, Murray MJ. *Clinical Anesthesiology*. 2nd ed. New York, NY: McGraw-Hill; 2002. Figure 4-10B.)

the bobbin to stick to the wall of the flowmeter. This would not allow you to accurately know what the actual flow would be.

The term *variable orifice* is also used. All that means is that the tube is *tapered* inside, being narrow at the bottom and gradually increasing in diameter toward the top. The *annular ring* is the little circular space that is between the indicator (bobbin) and the inside wall of the flowmeter; this is where the gas actually passes around the bobbin. The gas flows up the tube and causes the bobbin to travel with it until the pressure of the upward force of the gas is equal to the gravitational force on the bobbin (Figure 5-2).

At low flows, the gas flow is related to the viscosity of the gas and is smoother and laminar around the bobbin; at higher flows, the flow is related to the density of the gas and is turbulent. At higher altitudes (lower atmospheric pressure), the flowmeters read lower than actual flow.

At the top of each glass tube is a stopper that sticks down into view to keep the indicator or bobbin from rising out of the operator's sight behind the front panel of the machine (Figure 5-3).

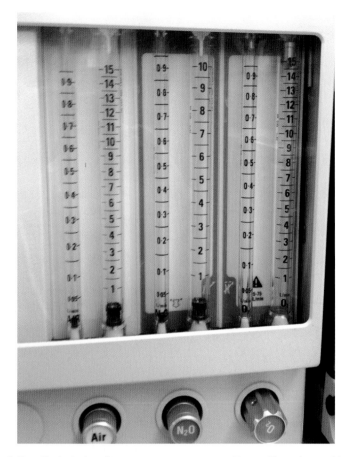

Figure 5-3 ▪ Typical glass flowmeters seen on many Datex-Ohmeda machines. Note the stoppers for bobbins at top of Thorpe tubes; with the oxygen flowmeter turned completely to maximum, the oxygen flowmeter is not easy to see.

The indicator will be either a bobbin shape or a ball. Some of them rotate while in use and may be colored differently along the outside so you can see the rotation. Some are stationary. If you want to be extremely precise in your flow, you should read the flow along the scale at the top of a bobbin or at the middle of a ball float.

Many machines have two flowmeters for at least oxygen and nitrous oxide that are in series. One is for fine measurements of 1 L/min flow, and the other takes over at flows of over 1 L/min (Figure 5-4).

Some anesthesia machines have digital flowmeters, where you do not see the actual flowmeter but only numbers on a screen. Still other modern machines have "virtual" flowmeters with an electronic representation of a

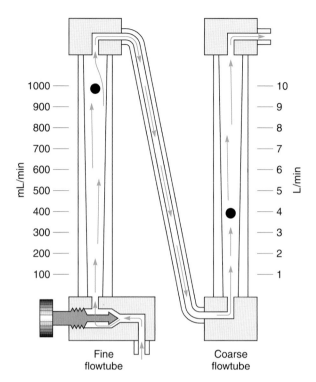

Figure 5-4 ▪ Two-tube flowmeter in series, enabling fine adjustments of low flow. (Reproduced with permission from Morgan GE, Mikhail MS, Murray MJ. *Clinical Anesthesiology*. 4th ed. New York, NY: McGraw-Hill; 2006. Figure 4-10A.)

flowmeter that is controlled with standard-looking knobs or touch pad buttons. An example of a machine such as this is the Draeger Apollo. Anesthesia machines with such digital or electronic flow readouts still (in most cases) have an old-fashioned glass flowmeter somewhere in view on the machine (Figure 5-5). This backup flowmeter is always "on," so you do not have to activate it in case your electronic screen stops working. Because it is only one flowmeter, not three, it measures the cumulative flow of *all* flowmeters that are in use.

At the top of all three flowmeters is the common manifold. This is where all three gases meet and continue their travel through the anesthesia machine. It is not visible unless the front panel is removed. It can be a site where leaks occur (more on that later).

Keep in mind that similar to vaporizers, flowmeters are specifically designed for each gas. If somehow a flowmeter tube was switched from one gas to another, the reading would be inaccurate.

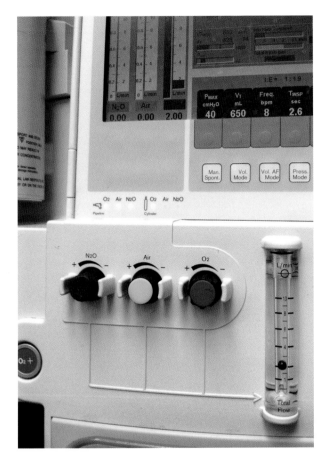

Figure 5-5 ■ "Virtual" or electronic readout flowmeters on the Draeger Apollo. Note the glass flowmeter to the right, which is the cumulative flow of all three gases, for use in case digital display is lost. Notice the protective guards around the control knobs, the fluting of the oxygen control knob, and the standard Draeger sequence of gases.

HAZARDS OF FLOWMETERS

Unrecognized Flow

What we mean by this is that a flowmeter may be on and you do not see that it is on. The knob could have been bumped by something despite the guard surrounding it and changed flow either up or down.

Another example is when the bobbin or ball is at the very top of the tube because the flowmeter has been turned up all the way for whatever reason. The anesthetist may not recognize this because the bobbin can be very unnoticeable at the very top. Consequently, there will be an unknown reason for incredibly high FGF or unexplained abnormal inspired oxygen concentration on the next anesthetic done with that machine. The authors have seen an instance of this when the air flowmeter was on full force and was not detected until an anesthetic was begun using that machine. The very high flow rates caused abnormally high tidal volumes and peak airway pressures that could not be explained until the error was discovered. This was a few years ago on a machine that did not have fresh gas compensation, so changes in FGF influenced tidal volumes (fresh gas compensation and decoupling are covered in the section on ventilators; see Figure 5-3).

Flowmeter Sequence, Leaks, and Hypoxia Risk

Every anesthesia general textbook for the past three decades or so probably has a diagram of how hypoxia can occur from flowmeter sequence and leaks. It has been shown that the best place for oxygen to be is the furthest downstream in relation to gas flow travel. This means that as you look at the front of an anesthesia machine, the flow of gas in the area of the flowmeters goes from left to right. So, oxygen is on the extreme right of the flowmeter section as a safety feature in case there were flowmeter glass cracks, breakage, or leaks in a flowmeter or in the manifold that connects them all.

Let's say there was a leak in the flowmeter of one or the other of the two gases besides oxygen on the machine. Let's also assume that the only flowmeter we are using is the oxygen flowmeter. Because the leak is upstream of oxygen, some oxygen would travel upstream and escape through the crack or leak, and some would travel downstream. Our total FGF would decrease but not our FiO_2 that is delivered to the patient.

Now let us look at another example. If there were a leak in either the air or nitrous oxide flowmeters and we were using that flowmeter, some of that gas would escape through the leak, and some would flow downstream. Because our oxygen flowmeter is downstream, we will not lose any significant FiO_2 because the portion of the upstream gas from the broken flowmeter would cause the oxygen to travel downstream with it. Usually when one small body of water joins a larger body of water, there is no retrograde flow; rather, all the newly added water goes downstream with the rest of the flow.

If our oxygen flowmeter was in the left or middle positions, we would lose oxygen concentration through a leak no matter where the leak was because it would travel either way, following the path of least resistance, and escape through the leak site.

The accompanying diagram we have included is based on the work of Edmond Eger and others who demonstrated that hypoxia was more likely if oxygen was *not* at the extreme right in flowmeter sequence (Figure 5-6). Dr. Eger's name may not be recognized by newer generations of anesthesiologists, but he

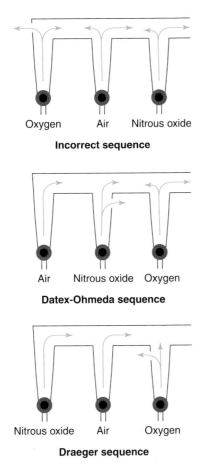

Oxygen   Air   Nitrous oxide

Incorrect sequence

Air   Nitrous oxide   Oxygen

Datex-Ohmeda sequence

Nitrous oxide   Air   Oxygen

Draeger sequence

Figure 5-6 ▪ Classic diagram of importance of flowmeter sequence in hypoxia prevention; note the different sequence of gases of the Datex-Ohmeda versus the Draeger machine, but both have oxygen at the end of the sequence. (Reproduced with permission from Morgan GE, Mikhail MS, Murray MJ. *Clinical Anesthesiology*. 4th ed. New York, NY: McGraw-Hill; 2006. Figure 4-11.)

is one of the giants of anesthesiology upon whose shoulders we all stand. He has made enormous contributions to the understanding of anesthetic uptake and distribution, among many other things.

Oxygen–Nitrous Oxide Proportioning

Built into anesthesia machines are several "fail-safes" to help us not deliver a hypoxic mixture to our patients. Part of these fail-safes has to do with flowmeters. We include them in a dedicated chapter on fail-safe mechanisms.

COMMON GAS OUTLET

After gas flow leaves the flowmeters, flowing through the rest of the low-pressure system, it travels to the vaporizers, which are discussed in detail in another Chapter 6. The end of the low-pressure system is the common gas outlet (Figure 5-7). This is the interface between the pneumatic system of the anesthesia machine and the ventilatory system of the machine. Think of the pneumatic system as the section of the machine that deals with obtaining and regulating the gases, combines them into what concentrations we want at what volume per minute, and adds our vaporized inhalational anesthetic agent to that mixture.

Most young anesthesiologists have probably never seen the common gas outlet of their machine because on modern machines, it is often integrated inside the machine. However, some modern machines do have a common gas outlet that is really a spur line from the actual common gas outlet. The visible outlet is not the actual one that connects our two sections together. But on older machines (those built up to about the end of the 1990s), the common gas outlet was placed in an external position with an external hose (thick so it could not be kinked) that connected the pneumatic and ventilatory systems. The hose could be disconnected from the outlet itself so the external common gas outlet could serve several other purposes. A Bain circuit could be hooked up there, so one could use nitrous oxide and inhalational agents through the Bain circuit. The low-pressure leak test was performed from there. If a catastrophic leak occurred in the ventilator, one could attach a bag valve mask to the outlet and deliver inhaled anesthetics, like with the Bain circuit. For that matter, these same functions can be done on any machine with a common gas outlet.

AUXILIARY FLOWMETER

Many anesthesia machines now have a built-in auxiliary oxygen flowmeter. It is located on the side of the machine above the circle circuit. It resembles the kind of flowmeter that is usually attached to a wall source, not like the oxygen, nitrous oxide, and air flowmeters you think of on an anesthesia machine. The maximum flow is 10 L/min. It is very convenient for delivering supplemental oxygen to patients who are undergoing a regional or neuraxial anesthetic or monitored anesthesia care. Other uses are limited only by the clinician's imagination. Many use it to insufflate oxygen through a fiberoptic bronchoscope during awake intubations, which serves to not only supply oxygen to the patient but also blow secretions or blood away from the tip of the bronchoscope. Keep in mind that some auxiliary flowmeters are designed to only

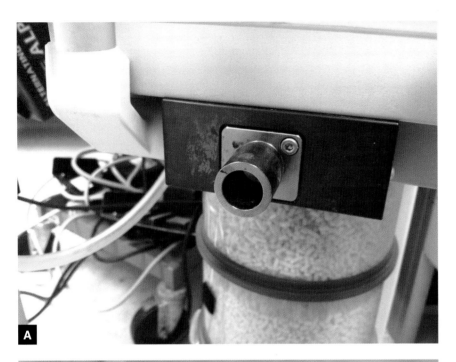

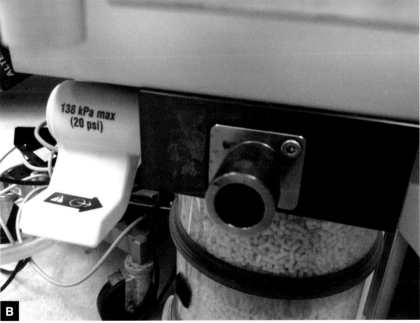

Figure 5-7 ■ (**A**) Common gas outlet on a Datex-Ohmeda Aestiva machine. (**B**) Note that switch must be engaged downward to open the gas outlet.

use a wall (pipeline) source of oxygen and will not function if you are using cylinders as your source of oxygen.

CONCLUSION

It is our hope that you now know more about flowmeters and the low-pressure system than before. Please remember, though, that the high-, intermediate-, and low-pressure systems are not individual sections of the machine as much as they are a way to divide, by the variable of pressure, a means of simplifying for us the workings inside an anesthesia machine.

VAPORIZERS | 6

KEYWORDS

- vaporizer types
- vaporizer safety features

Vaporizers are one of our interfaces with the anesthesia machine. We continually adjust them throughout each case we do. But do we really know what we are doing each time we move the dial?

Vaporizers are very complicated on the inside, much more than they may look to us. Inside each one there are things going on that pertain to gas laws, specific heat, vapor pressure, and all that stuff from chemistry we thought we would never see again. They are also categorized by certain qualities that may not make sense to us at first.

In this chapter, we will discuss how a vaporizer works, what each phrase in its classification means, and the hazards of vaporizers.

CHEMISTRY AND PHYSICS

Think about a can of gasoline. When it is open, you can smell the fumes emanating from the can. Another name for the fumes would be *vapor*. The fumes we smell are not a "gas" (three-letter word, not the short word for gasoline). A true "gas" is a chemical that has already reached its boiling point in the setting in which it finds itself. Oxygen, carbon dioxide, nitrogen, and so on are true "gases" in our environment because they exist at a temperature above their boiling points. That is why it is incorrect (but nevertheless common) to refer to inhalational agents as "gas" because they are not true gases at the temperature of an operating room (OR); they exist in a state below their boiling points. (Desflurane at room temperature is *almost* at its boiling point, however). The only commonly used "gases" found in an anesthesia machine are oxygen, air, and nitrous oxide.

Now think about a can of gasoline on a hot day. Gas cans nowadays are made out of plastic, not metal like in the past. On a hot day, a full can of gasoline can actually expand and deform itself. This is because the gasoline fumes, or *vapors,* are exerting a pressure against the sides of the gas can. This is called, simply enough, *vapor pressure.* This is an example of how above every liquid in a closed container, there exists a vapor pressure. In this situation, the vapor pressure is enough to distend the sides of the plastic can.

The molecules of hydrocarbons that make up what we call gasoline are leaving the surface of the liquid and floating up into the above space while at the same time molecules of gasoline are settling back down into the liquid from the vapor in the space above. The liquid and vapor are in *equilibrium* with each other.

A liquid and a vapor in an enclosed space will always find its own equilibrium (Figure 6-1). The amount of substance that is in liquid versus vapor phase in an enclosed container varies with temperature. For instance, on a day when it's 90°F, our can of gasoline has more molecules in a vapor phase than it would at 70°F (and therefore has a higher vapor pressure, thus distending the closed can). At 30°F, there would be less gasoline in a vapor phase still. There is the same amount of molecules of gasoline at all three temperatures, but the vapor pressure changes with changes in temperature because as the temperature increases, there is a shift to relatively more gasoline existing as a vapor than at lower temperatures.

So what does all this have to do with turning on the sevoflurane? There are things inside vaporizers that deal with the above concepts. Even the material that vaporizers are made of is important in ensuring an accurate delivery of what you dial in; more on all this to follow.

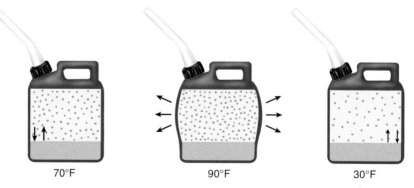

70°F   90°F   30°F

Figure 6-1 ▪ Notice at 90°F, there are more molecules in vapor form than at 70°F, and at 30°F, there are less molecules in vapor form than at 70°F. Also notice how the gasoline can at 90°F has expanded its walls—because more molecules are in vapor form, the vapor pressure is higher.

CLASSIFICATION OF VAPORIZERS

The modern vaporizer is classified as follows: variable bypass, agent specific, flow over, temperature compensated, and out of circuit. Each one of these phrases means something that you need to know about vaporizers (Figure 6-2).

Variable Bypass

When you adjust the knob of a vaporizer, you are *varying* how much of your fresh gas flow (FGF) (that you have dialed in from your flowmeters) goes into the vapor chamber versus how much *bypasses* the vapor chamber, thereby controlling how much of your FGF is exposed to your inhalational agent (and picks up the anesthetic vapor) and how much of your FGF goes straight through the vaporizer without picking up any vapor.

Agent Specific

Vaporizers for the past several decades have been designed to be *agent specific*, meaning that a certain vaporizer is constructed and calibrated to deliver a certain anesthetic agent based on qualities such as its vapor pressure, at a range of ambient room temperatures found in ORs, throughout a wide range of FGF rates (from 250 cc/min to 15 L/min). We all know that vaporizers are labeled and colored a certain color for each agent. In fact, we probably rely more on the vaporizer *color* than reading the label.

Up until the early 1990s, there was no safeguard to ensure that the correct liquid was poured into the correct vaporizer. Vaporizers back then had a simple screw-on lid that you opened and filled the vaporizer through. If you weren't paying attention or were in a room with the lights dimmed, it would have been easy to mistakenly pour the incorrect agent into the incorrect vaporizer (especially with halothane and enflurane—one was colored orange-red and the other reddish orange!). We will discuss the implications of misfilling a vaporizer later on in the chapter.

Of course, now there are various fail-safes to guard against misfilling a vaporizer. We are all familiar with the collars that are on bottles of liquid agent. The collars have tabs that will only allow the correct attachment that will fit the refilling inlet of the vaporizer in question. Draeger uses a funnel-type system, and Ohmeda uses a "key" siphon system; both systems are agent specific and manufacturer specific.

Flow Over

When you turn the vaporizer control knob and *vary* the amount of FGF that *bypasses* the vapor chamber, a portion of the FGF is directed into the vapor

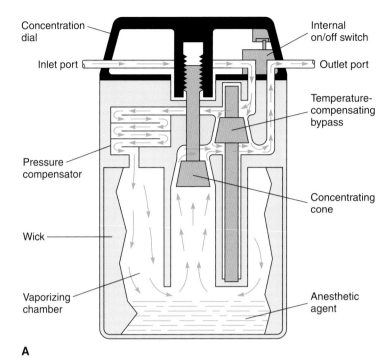

Concentration dial

Inlet port

Internal on/off switch

Outlet port

Temperature-compensating bypass

Pressure compensator

Concentrating cone

Wick

Vaporizing chamber

Anesthetic agent

A

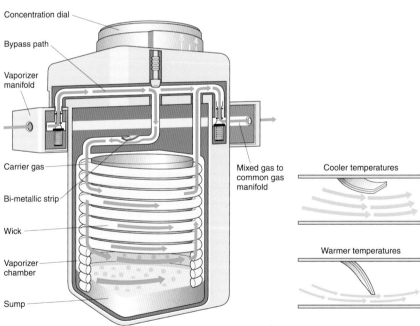

Concentration dial

Bypass path

Vaporizer manifold

Carrier gas

Bi-metallic strip

Wick

Vaporizer chamber

Sump

Mixed gas to common gas manifold

Cooler temperatures

Warmer temperatures

B

Figure 6-2 ▪ Schematic of agent-specific variable-bypass vaporizers. (**A**) Draeger Vapor 19.n. (**B**) Datex-Ohmeda Tec 7. (Reproduced with permission from Morgan GE, Mikhail MS, Murray MJ. *Clinical Anesthesiology*. 4th ed. New York, NY: McGraw-Hill; 2006. Figure 4-19A, B.)

chamber. There, it *flows over* the top of the liquid agent, picking up the vapor that is above the liquid.

Older vaporizers were called "bubble through" because the FGF would actually bubble through the liquid agent from the bottom of the chamber, similar to blowing bubbles in a glass with a drinking straw. The bubbles with their great amount of surface area would pick up molecules of the anesthetic agent in that manner.

It is easy to see by the size of a vaporizer that there is not much surface area for the liquid anesthetics in their chamber. There might be enough surface area of the liquid agent for enough vapor to be picked up at low FGF, but how about when you have sevoflurane at 3% and 6 L/min FGF? There is definitely not enough surface area for accurate delivery at such a rate. Enter the wick.

Inside vaporizers there are wicks, analogous to lantern wicks, along the sides of the vaporizing chamber that absorb the liquid agent. By capillary action, the liquid is spread out all over the wick. This greatly increases the surface area of the liquid, so more vapor is picked up by our FGF. The wicks make the sides of the vaporizing chamber a surface area for the liquid in addition to merely the top of the liquid in the bottom of the vaporizer.

Temperature Compensation

As we saw earlier by observing our gasoline can at various temperatures, vapor pressure is dependent on temperature. The higher the ambient temperature, the more the vapor a liquid will have above it in a closed container and vice versa.

So what happens in the OR when the room temperature may be high in a pediatric room and cold in the heart room? Even in the range of temperatures seen in ORs, the amount of vapor above our liquid anesthetic agent in the vaporizer will differ from room to room because of temperature differences. There will be more agent in the vapor phase in the pediatric room versus the heart room. This would influence accurate delivery of how much agent we have dialed in if there were no *compensation* for *temperature* differences.

In addition to differences in room temperature, the vaporizer needs to compensate for changes in temperature inside the vaporizing chamber as a direct result of the vaporizing process. Vaporization of a liquid takes energy. That energy comes from the heat of the liquid that is vaporizing. This is called the *latent heat of vaporization*. So as we provide an anesthetic, the temperature of our liquid agent is decreasing because it is losing heat in the process of vapor formation.

Therefore, we have two potential causes of temperature problems in vaporizers: ambient temperature changes and loss of heat from vaporization. Now let's say that our vaporizers were designed to work at 25°C. If the room was warmer, the output of anesthetic from the vaporizer would be more than we have dialed in; conversely, if the room was colder, our agent output would be less than what we want. On top of that, we are also losing heat from the process of vaporization of our liquid agent.

Fortunately, there are means of *temperature compensation*. There is a device inside a vaporizer that changes shape or length with changes in ambient temperature. Think about junior high school science class. You may have studied about how a thermostat on the wall has a bimetallic strip inside it that changes shape or length in response to changes in room temperature. That is how a thermostat knows when to turn on or shut off.

Some vaporizers have a rod that changes length in response to temperature changes and is precisely calibrated so that it will allow more or less FGF into the vapor chamber, automatically as needed. Other manufacturers have a precisely calibrated bimetallic strip that either blocks FGF into the vaporizing chamber or allows more FGF into the chamber based on ambient temperature. This keeps the output of the vaporizer the same whether you are using it in the pediatric room or the heart room (Figure 6-3).

There is another form of temperature compensation. Vaporizers are made of metals that conduct heat well, so the vaporizer structure itself draws heat from the room, causing less of a change in liquid agent temperature as energy (and therefore heat) is lost by the process of vaporization.

Some vaporizing systems are computerized and are programmed to inject more or less vapor into the FGF depending on ambient temperature similar to fuel injection in an automobile. These vaporizers, of course,

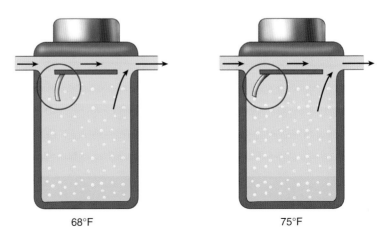

68°F   75°F

Figure 6-3 ▪ The bimetallic strip at 68°F lets more of the fresh gas flow enter the vapor chamber compared with the bimetallic strip at 75°F, where more agent is in the vapor phase. This calibrated strip keeps the vaporizer output the same for different room temperatures.

require electricity, but the simpler ones we have been discussing do not. (That is one of the great things about standard vaporizers—they work without electricity. Later we will discuss what happens to an anesthesia machine when the power goes out.)

Out of Circuit

In the past, some vaporizers actually were attached to the circle system instead of being placed upstream of the circuit like modern anesthesia machines are configured. These vaporizers were more inaccurate than current types but nevertheless were used to a great extent and are still used in veterinary practice and in developing countries. One problem with the in-circuit vaporizers is that they can accumulate moisture from the patient's exhalation to an extent that there can be a layer of water above the liquid anesthetic agent, greatly decreasing vapor output. Another problem was because some in-circuit vaporizers were not locked onto the machine, they could be tipped over (tipping is discussed next).

▌ HAZARDS OF VAPORIZERS

Tipping

If a vaporizer containing liquid anesthetic agent falls on its side or is even tipped too much, liquid agent will find its way into the bypass pathway. When the vaporizer is used next, the FGF will vaporize the agent in the bypass tubing, subjecting the patient to extremely high or even lethal levels of agent vapor. It only takes one milliliter of liquid agent to produce 200 mL of anesthetic vapor, so you can see the danger if the bypass chamber was flooded with liquid agent.

If a vaporizer is tipped, it should be drained of all liquid agent. Then the vaporizer should be turned on (after being mounted back where it is supposed to be on the machine) a small degree and flushed with high FGF until no agent is detectable by gas monitoring.

This is one reason why vaporizers are connected so securely to an anesthesia machine. Tipping frequently occurs when a vaporizer is being moved from one machine to another, so some vaporizers have a "T" transport mode on the dial, which effectively blocks any liquid from reaching the bypass area.

Overfilling

Overfilling was a problem in the past with older designs of vaporizers. If the vaporizer was overfilled, a situation similar to tipping occurred when liquid agent got into the bypass chamber, leading to a greatly increased vapor concentration of anesthetic. Current vaporizers are designed now as to prohibit or minimize the chance of overfilling.

Simultaneous Administration

Our inhalational anesthetics are very potent; even at 1 minimum alveolar concentration (MAC), they can cause hemodynamic instability. It is not hard to realize that if two agents were being given simultaneously, overdosing the patient would be easy. Fortunately, there are mechanisms that block us from mistakenly turning on more than one vaporizer at the same time.

There is an *interlock* system for all modern vaporizers. When the vaporizer dial is turned on, the locking mechanism activates. Draeger and Ohmeda have different designs of interlocking devices. (Of course, it does not matter that they are incompatible because vaporizers will not fit on the other company's machine.)

The system for Ohmeda machines is simple and visible (Figure 6-4). When the vaporizer is turned on, pins on the sides of the vaporizer pop out. The vaporizer next to it has pins adjacent to the pins that have now popped out and are pushed in by the first pins. This locks the other vaporizer because the pins must be free to extend to turn on the vaporizer.

Misfilling

One would have to deliberately work to defeat modern agent-specific filling systems (Figure 6-5). Putting a less potent agent into a vaporizer designed for an agent of higher potency (e.g., sevoflurane into an isoflurane vaporizer) would result in delivering *less* of an anesthetic dose than desired. Putting a higher potency agent into a vaporizer designed for a less potent agent

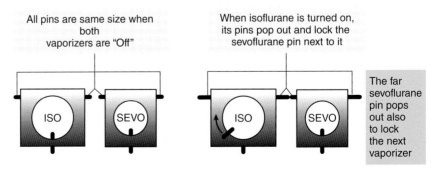

Figure 6-4 ▪ Datex Ohmeda Tec vaporizer interlock system viewed from above.

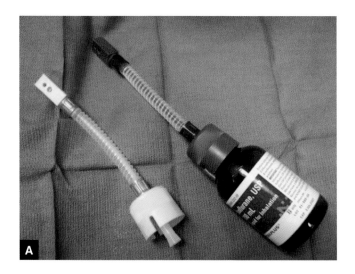

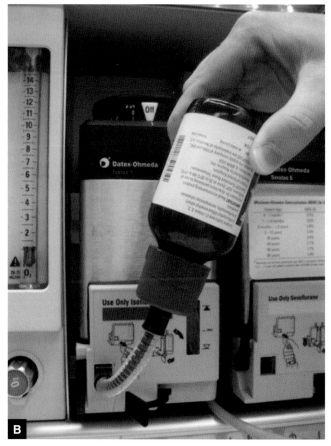

Figure 6-5 ▪ (**A**) and (**B**) Agent-specific filling siphons for Datex-Ohmeda vaporizers.

(e.g., isoflurane into a sevoflurane vaporizer) would result in delivering *more* anesthetic than desired.

However, when giving the example of sevoflurane versus isoflurane, the difference would be about 1 MAC versus ½ MAC. A vigilant anesthetist would see that the patient's response to the supposed amount of agent was not what is should be, whether the patient was getting too much or too little inhalational agent, in regards to vital signs, movement, bispectral index (BIS), and so on. If your gas monitor is reading sevoflurane when you think you are using isoflurane, you need to investigate.

What this all boils down to is that if you are using isoflurane or sevoflurane in the wrong vaporizer, it should be readily and quickly discovered. That was not the case in the past, when monitoring was not as sophisticated. Respiratory monitoring of agent concentration and type has been in common since the mid to late 1980s. Before then, delivery of the wrong agent was a much more serious and potentially common occurrence.

The vaporizers in the past were agent specific, and similar to the ones in use today, there was no agent-specific filling system. You simply unscrewed the lid and poured in whatever. As mentioned earlier, halothane's label color was red, and enfluranes's was orange. If you misfiled either one of those agents into the wrong vaporizer, you would have serious problems.

The MAC of halothane is 0.75%. The MAC of enflurane is 1.7%. So if you put halothane into an enflurane vaporizer and turned the dial to deliver around 2%, you were delivering in excess of 2 MAC of halothane. That is a lot of halothane—enough for myocardial depression. Halothane is a very strong myocardial depressant, and you could get into a lot trouble quickly when you were in the 2+ MAC range. Now complicate the scenario by not having respiratory gas monitoring to give you the dosage and identity of the agent.

Consider misfilling a standard vaporizer with desflurane. Fortunately, the connections between the bottle and vaporizer would keep a person from accidentally misfilling desflurane into a standard vaporizer. If it did happen, though, a potentially lethal amount of desflurane would be vaporized and administered to the patient.

Leaks

When some vaporizers are filled, various plugs and caps must be closed. Failure to replace or properly tighten these pieces will result in a leak when the vaporizer is turned on. The leak will cause a relative *underdosing* of the patient seen in the respiratory gas monitoring data. The leak may or may not be detectable by smell—it can be too small to generate enough odor or other odors in the OR may mask the presence of agent in the air.

Low Agent

Unlike a desflurane vaporizer, regular vaporizers do not alarm when they are getting close to empty. Vaporizers should be checked before each case to see if they need to be refilled. As more and more electronics are introduced into vaporizer design, low-volume alarms will become more common.

Vaporizer Left On

At some time in your career, you will start to preoxygenate a patient for induction and subsequently see that a vaporizer is turned on, either by the patient complaining of or reacting to the odor, by seeing agent on your gas monitor, or by seeing that the vaporizer dial is on. Invariably, this occurs because the last patient in the room was transported to the recovery room or unit "asleep" and the agent was therefore left on and not turned off. Again, vaporizers should be checked before each case not only to check if they need to be refilled but also to ensure that they are off and to make sure they are closed properly. Checking vaporizers is part of the standard machine check-out.

Pumping

Pumping was more of a concern years ago before end-tidal and inspiratory agent monitoring was commonplace. The pumping effect could increase the concentration of agent enough to be clinically significant. The clinician would be "flying blind," not knowing he or she was giving more agent than was thought without the use of agent monitoring. In addition, older machines did not have check valves between the ventilator and the vaporizer to decrease the intensity of the backpressure.

When the ventilator cycles, it causes some retrograde pressure that travels to the vaporizer. This causes a momentary increase in vaporizer output. The retrograde pressure causes a temporary halt in flow coming out of the vapor chamber. When the pressure is released, the volume of gas in the vapor chamber travels out its normal path but also travels backward up to the bypass chamber. There are two paths that momentarily have saturated gas, and this is what increases concentration. Figure 6-6 illustrates the retrograde pressure that causes the pumping effect when the oxygen flush is activated. You will see a quick jump of the flowmeter bobbins. Modern machines have one-way check valves between the ventilator and the vaporizers to decrease the backward pressure changes that cause pumping.

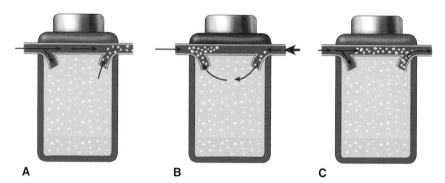

A   **B**   **C**

Figure 6-6 ■ Vaporizer pumping diagram. (**A**) Normal vaporizer function. (**B**) Momentary backpressure from the ventilator causing vapor to flow in a retrograde manner into the bypass chamber. (**C**) Vapor flowing through the bypass chamber, joining with the regular amount of anesthetic agent vapor.

Mislabeled Vaporizer

There has been at least one report of a vaporizer that was mislabeled. Its built-in plastic parts were purple, the color for isoflurane. Its agent-specific filling apparatus was for isoflurane. But the front cap on the vaporizer was labeled "sevoflurane." In fact, it had been in use in a busy OR for some time without notice (Figure 6-7). This illustrates how, at least for vaporizers, we rely more on color than labeling.

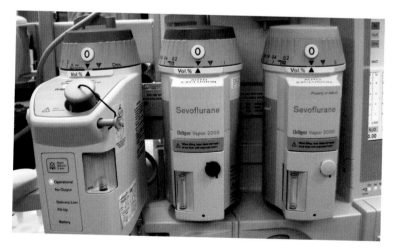

Figure 6-7 ■ Mislabeled isoflurane vaporizer; notice the purple colors on the center vaporizer even though it is labeled sevoflurane; the vaporizer was, in fact, an isoflurane vaporizer that had come with a front plate labeled "sevoflurane."

DESFLURANE VAPORIZER

You may have noticed that we have not discussed desflurane very much so far in this chapter. Desflurane and its vaporizer are very much different than the vaporizers we have been discussing (those for isoflurane, sevoflurane, and even halothane and enflurane).

By now you should at least understand the basics of a regular vaporizer, what is inside it, and how it works. You should even be able to draw a simple diagram of how one works. Desflurane vaporizers are very different looking on the inside, however. A schematic diagram of a desflurane vaporizer would be very confusing unless perhaps you were an electrical engineer. Most of what is inside a desflurane vaporizer is electronic. Desflurane requires a very special device to accurately deliver its vapor; the vaporizer requires electricity because it produces heat and pressure inside in order to properly function.

Desflurane is very volatile. It has a very low boiling point (23.5°C, or 74.3°F). If you pour a little desflurane on the metal shelf of an anesthesia machine, you can watch the liquid disappear quickly. Because desflurane is so volatile, a small change in temperature will greatly increase vapor. A temperature of 74.3°F is a little warm for an OR, but it is still close to what the ambient temperature of most ORs would be.

Because even small variations in room temperature would cause large changes in the amount of desflurane vapor above liquid desflurane in a closed container, the designers of the desflurane vaporizer decided to take out the variable of temperature. The vaporizer is therefore heated to 39°C, so changes in room temperature will have no bearing on how much desflurane is in vapor phase.

But remember that the boiling point of desflurane is 23.5°C. So why doesn't *all* the desflurane that is heated to 39°C in its special vaporizer become vapor? This is because in addition to heating the desflurane, the special vaporizer also *pressurizes* the desflurane. Liquids under pressure have higher boiling points. The designers, if they wanted to keep the temperature of the desflurane in its vaporizer steady, needed to pressurize it so it wouldn't all boil away at a little above room temperature. The pressure inside the desflurane vaporizer is twice that of sea level (2 atm, or 200 kilopascals). The need for heating and pressurizing is why the desflurane vaporizer needs electricity.

There is another difference between the desflurane vaporizers and standard vaporizers. A desflurane vaporizer is not a "flow-over" type like we discussed earlier in the chapter. Actually, the desflurane vapor is injected into the FGF.

If you turn a bottle of desflurane upside down, nothing comes out. That is because the bottle has a spring-loaded valve that must be pushed in to open the bottle. This keeps desflurane from vaporizing while you unscrew the lid and prepare to fill the desflurane vaporizer. When you seat the bottle into the filling port, the valve is opened, and the desflurane empties.

ALADIN CASSETTE

The Datex-Ohmeda ADU anesthesia machine has a novel kind of vaporizer. Instead of a separate vaporizer for each agent, there are "cassettes," or containers in the appropriate color for each agent. There is a built-in slot on the ADU machine where the cassette is placed to deliver that specific agent. Each cassette has a handle and a trigger device to change cassettes easily in seconds even during a case (Figure 6-8).

The cassette itself is simply a pan that houses the liquid agent. If it is tipped, there is no problem because the bypass chamber itself is in the built-in slot in the machine where you put the cassette. Each cassette has a magnetic identity strip on the back of it that is read by the detectors in the slot. A central processing unit (CPU) in the slot knows what agent is being used and tailors the amount of FGF that goes into the cassette.

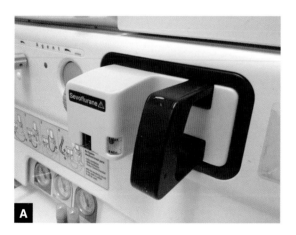

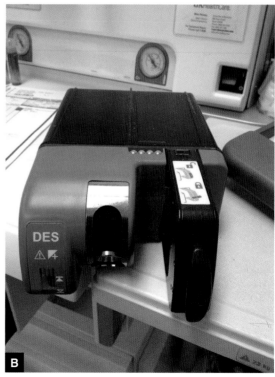

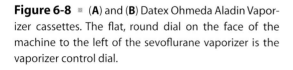

Figure 6-8 ■ (**A**) and (**B**) Datex Ohmeda Aladin Vaporizer cassettes. The flat, round dial on the face of the machine to the left of the sevoflurane vaporizer is the vaporizer control dial.

There is no dial on the cassette to control concentration. Changes in vapor concentration are done via a dial on the front of the ADU, with the readout on the video screen on the ADU machine. When a cassette is switched out for another, the electronic control changes automatically on the screen also, and you must remember to adjust the agent output accordingly. The delivery is as accurate as for regular vaporizers because ambient temperature, FGF, and what amount of FGF to divert into the cassette are handled by the CPU. This type of vaporizer *needs* electricity to work.

MAQUET VAPORIZERS

Maquet vaporizers are specialized for use only on Maquet anesthesia machines. They are a type of injection vaporizer. Part of the FGF is diverted into the liquid agent chamber, pressurizing it. The increase in pressure causes a calibrated amount of agent to go through an injection port back into the FGF pathway. These vaporizers are agent-specific, out-of-circuit vaporizers but do not require temperature compensation because of how they work. They require electricity to work.

FUTURE VAPORIZERS

Already the major manufacturers are offering vaporizers that require an outside power source to function. The benefit of such a vaporizer is that output of the vaporizer will automatically adjust depending on its FGF rate. For instance, with a regular sevoflurane vaporizer, if you have a high FGF while delivering 3% sevoflurane and then reduce the FGF, the concentration of sevoflurane in the circuit will decrease. The reason is that when you decrease the FGF, it takes longer to equilibrate all the volume of your circuit, so even though there is the same *concentration* of sevoflurane being released by the vaporizer, there is less *volume* of sevoflurane coming out of the vaporizer to fill up the circuit. Equilibration will happen with low FGF, but it takes longer.

New vaporizers will automatically correct for that by sensing devices in the inspiratory and expiratory limbs that will ensure the desired concentration that you have dialed will stay the same with changes in FGF. The days of the simple nonelectric vaporizer may be numbered.

One new kind of "vaporizer" is called an *anesthetic conserving device* (ACD). It is not a vaporizer in the sense that we have been discussing but rather an inhalational anesthetic delivery device. A liquid anesthetic agent is delivered by a syringe pump to a chamber that has a rod made of porous material. The rod soaks up the agent. The FGF of the anesthesia machine or ventilator will vaporize the anesthetic agent from the rod, sending it to the patient.

On exhalation, a filter-like device (presumably close to the endotracheal tube) similar to a heat and moisture exchanger (HME) made of activated charcoal fibers absorbs the exhaled anesthetic. On the next inspiration, the activated charcoal releases most of its absorbed agent back into the patient. The output of liquid agent from the syringe pump is controlled by readouts of inspired and end-tidal agent.

Because a standard circle circuit that allows rebreathing is not required for this kind of agent conservation, the ACD has been considered for use with intensive care unit (ICU) type ventilators in a critical care setting for use in inhalational sedation. Some form of scavenger system will be needed because up to now ICU ventilators in general have no need for scavenging of waste gases.

CONCLUSION

We hope this chapter has taken some of the mystery out of exactly what happens inside an anesthesia vaporizer. Many highly skilled engineers, scientists, and physicians have worked on the most effective way to deliver anesthetic vapor over the years, and it is we and our patients who are the beneficiaries of their efforts. We should remember this whenever we turn on, adjust, or fill a vaporizer.

CIRCLE CIRCUIT | 7

The circle circuit is not a true circle in shape, of course. It is a circle in that it is a continuous loop that recycles gas and anesthetic agent from the patient. It is the end point of gas delivery to the patient. It all seems simple, but on second look, there are a lot of things that make the circle circuit possible. Some of them you may know about, but some you may *not* know about.

In this chapter, we will go from one end of the circle and back again, going all around the circuit to understand it. One part of the circle system, the carbon dioxide absorber, is discussed in its own chapter.

There are two important points that allow the circle circuit to work: one is that there is flow going only *one way* through it, and the other is that carbon dioxide is removed from the exhaled breath. The circle circuit has many parts, so we will discuss each one. We will start inside the machine and work our way around.

PARTS OF THE CIRCLE CIRCUIT

Fresh Gas Inlet

We will begin the journey at the fresh gas outlet (Figure 7-1). The fresh gas inlet is where the gas from the pneumatic part of the machine enters the circuit. It is really an extension of the common gas outlet that we discussed in

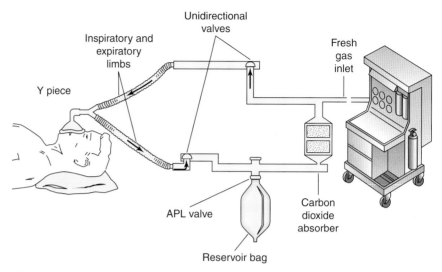

Figure 7-1 ▪ Major parts of the circle circuit. APL, adjustable pressure-limiting. (Reproduced with permission from Morgan GE, Mikhail MS, Murray MJ. *Clinical Anesthesiology*. 4th ed. New York, NY: McGraw-Hill; 2006. Figure 3-1.)

the chapter on the low-pressure pneumatic; kind of like a road that changes its name at an intersection, it is called the common gas outlet on one end and the fresh gas outlet on the other end. The fresh gas inlet can enter the circle at any place theoretically but almost always comes in upstream of the inspiratory unidirectional valve and downstream of the absorber (Figure 7-2).

Unidirectional Valves

Remember we said there is *one-way* flow through the circle. It is the unidirectional valves that make this so. The unidirectional valves are another part of the anesthesia machine that were designed simplistically and not overengineered to do their job. They require no electricity either.

The unidirectional valves are found at the start of the inspiratory and end of the expiratory limbs (Figure 7-3). The inspiratory valve allows flow toward the patient only with no flow back toward the machine. The expiratory valve allows flow away from the patient only with no flow back toward the patient. The valves are somewhat mirror images of the other. We will discuss how the inspiratory valve works first.

The valve consists of a flat plastic disk about the size of a 50 cent piece but thinner. On almost all machines, it is seated horizontally on a round, thin-walled valve seat. It is held in place by a spider-like looking cage over the top of the disk, and the whole assembly is under a clear plastic dome that is

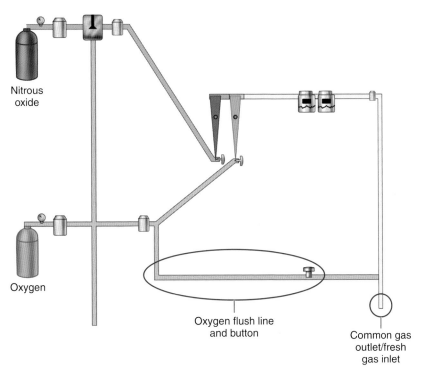

Nitrous
oxide

Oxygen

Oxygen flush line
and button

Common gas
outlet/fresh
gas inlet

Figure 7-2 ▪ Schematic of the common gas outlet at the end of pneumatic section of machine, becoming the fresh gas inlet at the start of the ventilatory section of the machine.

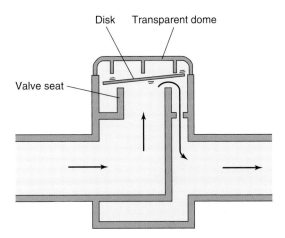

Disk   Transparent dome

Valve seat

Figure 7-3 ▪ A unidirectional valve. (Reproduced with permission from Morgan GE, Mikhail MS, Murray MJ. *Clinical Anesthesiology*. 4th ed. New York, NY: McGraw-Hill; 2006. Figure 3-9.)

visible from the operator's position. Flow going through the valve lifts the disk off its seat, allowing flow traveling in one direction. The instant that the flow is reversed (e.g., exhalation), the disk is pushed back on its round valve seat, thereby blocking flow.

The expiratory unidirectional valve works similarly. Expiratory flow is directed under the disk to lift it off its valve seat. The instant that reverse flow is detected, the disk is pushed back against its valve seat.

The valves are situated on the machine so that they can be clearly seen and inspected for proper function. They are also labeled either by name or by an arrow indicating flow travel. On some machines, such as the Datex-Ohmeda ADU, the unidirectional valves are mounted vertically and not horizontally. Their function is the same. Things can go wrong with unidirectional valves, and we will discuss that later in the chapter.

Inspiratory and Expiratory Ports

These are where the circle tubing connects to the machine. The ports are found immediately downstream of their respective unidirectional valves. The size of the ports is 22 mm. The ports stick out about 1.5 inches or so perpendicularly from their mounting to allow the circle limbs to slip on tightly. The ports are usually made out of metal. But sometimes they are made out of plastic (like the Draeger Apollo), are angled, and have a collar around them that can be loosened to direct the angled port in a different way. (These collars can be the site for leaks; more on this later.)

Circuit Tubing

Circuit tubing is made of plastic and is corrugated. The corrugations are there to decrease kinking and to allow the plastic tubing to bend easily. The tubing comes in adult and pediatric sizes. It is white in color compared with the blue color of stiffer critical care ventilator circuits. Because anesthesia circuit tubing is softer and more pliable than critical care ventilators, the actual tidal volume (TV) may not be what you think you dialed in initially. Gas is compressible, and the circuit tubing is expandable—you can often see it "wiggle" during a ventilatory cycle. This is more visible if the patient's peak airway pressure is high.

On older machines, this would often change the delivered TV to a significant degree. However, modern anesthesia ventilators have more sophisticated volume sensors in a feedback loop to deal with this wasted ventilation.

Y Piece

The Y piece is where the inspiratory and expiratory limbs of the circuit meet, and form a common pathway to the circuit–patient interface (e.g., facemask, endotracheal tube, or supraglottic device). It is the only part of the circle circuit where there is dead space, meaning there is rebreathing of gas containing carbon dioxide.

Of course, we say the circle circuit is all about rebreathing, but the carbon dioxide is eliminated in the course of rebreathing. With the Y piece, there is a small amount of gas that has carbon dioxide in it that is rebreathed because the gas at the end of expiration doesn't make it all the way out past the Y piece and down the expiratory limb. That small volume of carbon dioxide containing gas is still in the Y piece when inspiration begins. This is true for controlled or spontaneous ventilation.

Think about the volume of a Y piece. It is not very much when compared with an adult TV, but the dead space volume from the Y piece can be significant for neonates and can lead to hypercarbia in neonatal anesthesia. Y piece volumes can differ slightly depending on the shape and configuration of the circuits from different manufacturers, and there is a difference in volumes between adult and pediatric circuits.

The Y piece can also have adapters built into it to attach gas sampling lines and even temperature sensors for heated humidifiers.

Along with the Y piece, there is the "elbow," a small right angle connector whose main function is to redirect the circuit at its takeoff from the facemask, endotracheal tube, or supraglottic device. It is made to accept a 22-mm female adapter (facemask) or 15-mm male adapter (endotracheal tube, supraglottic device). The Y piece itself has the same connector size ability. Y pieces and elbows are prime candidates for disconnection locations.

Adjustable Pressure-Limiting Valve

This valve, more commonly known as the adjustable pressure-limiting (APL) or "pop-off" valve, is located downstream of the expiratory unidirectional valve. Its function may be familiar to most clinicians, but how it works is not well understood by most of us. Exactly what is happening when we turn the APL knob?

The APL valve is the interface between the circuit and the scavenger system (Figure 7-4). It controls the pressure in the circuit during manual or spontaneous ventilation with a circle circuit. When the APL is completely open, excess volume from the circuit is vented into the scavenger. (Remember that excess volume is related to whatever your fresh gas flow (FGF) is; what goes in must come out of the machine, either through the scavenger or through leaks somewhere else in the circuit such as a poorly sealed facemask.)

As you turn the APL knob clockwise, the APL valve opening gets smaller, so less of your excess volume goes into the scavenger. That is why it helps to

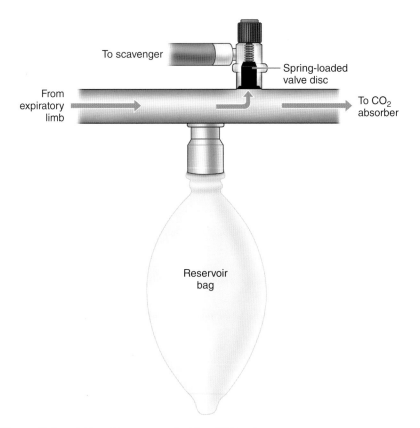

Figure 7-4 ▪ Adjustable pressure-limiting (APL) valve.

turn your APL knob closed whenever you have a difficult mask airway—more volume is available to you to try to squeeze into the patient's lungs. Turning the knob counterclockwise opens the valve. Some valves have knobs that click as they are adjusted, and some have numbers corresponding to the airway pressure at a specific setting.

There is a spring-loaded valve inside the APL housing. It may be a disk type valve, or it may be a type that is more like a water faucet, opening a valve seat as you turn the stem. There will also be a unidirectional disc valve similar to the inspiratory and expiratory valves that will prevent backpressure and subsequent barotrauma from the scavenger.

The APL valve is not part of the in-line path of the circle circuit but is more like a branch or sideline device that allows us to "pop off" excess volume (and therefore pressure) when we do not need it based on our clinical experience. It is bypassed totally when the ventilator is turned on. Excess gas from the ventilator is vented into the scavenger by another pathway.

As mentioned, the APL valve is located downstream of the expiratory unidirectional valve and is close to the reservoir bag. It could be placed in several different positions, but in this position, the excess gas is vented into the scavenger before it goes through the carbon dioxide absorber, saving absorbent because we aren't wasting our absorbing capacity on gas we are going to discard.

The location on the machine itself of the APL valve knob varies not only from manufacturer to manufacturer but also from model to model. In general, the knob is close to the reservoir bag because it ergonomically makes sense to have knob and bag close because the right hand is used for both. Some knobs are mounted horizontally, and some are mounted vertically.

Reservoir Bag

This is one of the most familiar components of an anesthesia machine, and even laypeople have seen a reservoir bag moving in and out on TV shows. It seems so simple; what else do we need to know about it except it is made of rubber and we squeeze it?

The bag allows us to manually ventilate the patient. It also allows us to monitor the patient's spontaneous ventilations. As the name suggests, the bag is also a *reservoir* for gas for the circuit. In addition, for some types of anesthesia ventilators, such as the Draeger piston drive machines, the reservoir bag is an integral part. FGF is diverted (decoupled) into the reservoir bag during inspiration. If you disconnected the bag on such a machine while using the ventilator, you would cause a big leak. For bellows-type ventilators, the reservoir bag plays no role; disconnecting the bag causes no leak or malfunction. We discuss this in more depth in Chapter 8 on anesthesia ventilators.

The bag connects to the machine by a swivel arm, either rigid or flexible like a gooseneck lamp. The bag connection is 22 mm female. This allows the bag to be attached to the anesthesia circuit to act like a lung to check the ventilator (but remember, taking off the bag will cause a leak on ventilators such as the Draeger Apollo).

The location of the bag in the circle is usually between the expiratory unidirectional valve and the carbon dioxide absorber. The bag's function is closely associated with that of the APL valve, as discussed previously. However, on some machines, the reservoir bag is found in different sites along the circle.

Bags are made from both latex and nonlatex material and come in adult (3-L volume), pediatric (1-L volume), and in-between (2-L volume) sizes.

Selector Switch

This switch merely acts like a stopcock to change flow from the bag and APL to the ventilator. It is important to remember that when switched from bag to ventilator, *the APL valve is bypassed*. The switch can be mechanical or electronic; going from bag to ventilator automatically turns on the ventilator and vice versa. Remember that with more sophisticated anesthesia ventilators that have pressure support mode along with volume control and pressure control, the reservoir bag is not part of the pressure support circuit even though the patient may be breathing spontaneously. The authors have seen episodes when a spontaneously breathing patient emerges from anesthesia while still on pressure support and is extubated, then goes into laryngospasm or obstructs, and no positive-pressure ventilation is produced from squeezing the reservoir bag *because* the selector switch *is still on ventilator/pressure support mode* (Figure 7-5).

Respirometer

This device measures the *volume* of each breath. Various kinds of volume meters are used in anesthesia machines. A vane anemometer (Figure 7-6) counts rotations of a pinwheel inside the circuit and calculates volume from how many rotations of the pinwheel occur per breath. Some use ultrasound as a measuring means. A hot wire anemometer is found on modern Draeger

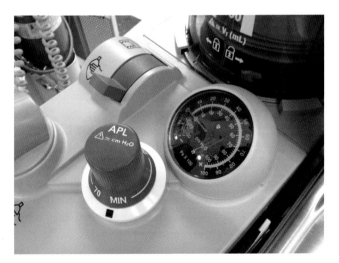

Figure 7-5 ▪ Selector switch of the Datex-Ohmeda Aestiva 5 machine. In addition to switching from the reservoir bag to the ventilator, it also turns on the ventilator. Also note the adjustable pressure-limiting valve and airway pressure gauge.

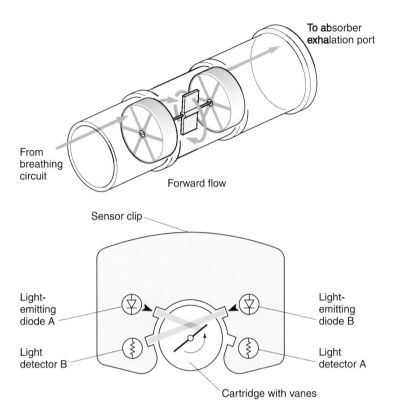

Figure 7-6 ▪ Vane anemometer. (Reproduced with permission from Morgan GE, Mikhail MS, Murray MJ. *Clinical Anesthesiology*. 4th ed. New York, NY: McGraw-Hill; 2006. Figure 4-24A.)

machines and has a heated wire in its lumen; it calculates TV by the drop in temperature of the heated wire as it is cooled by the gas flow. A variable-orifice respirometer (Figure 7-7) senses pressure changes across an orifice and calculates volume in that manner.

Yet another kind of respirometer is called a *D-Lite* (Figure 7-8). It uses a mainstream insert, not unlike a heat and moisture exchanger (HME), next to the Y piece. There are two pitot tubes inside the insert, each facing the opposite way. They measure both inspiratory and expiratory TV as a function of change in pressure during the ventilatory cycle (similar to the pitot tubes on airplanes measure airspeed). This system is found on the Datex-Ohmeda ADU. The D-Lite system is also used for respiratory gas monitoring. It comes in different sizes for adult and pediatric circle circuits.

Modern anesthesia machines have two sets of respirometers: one on the inspiratory side and one on the expiratory side of the circle circuit. In this way,

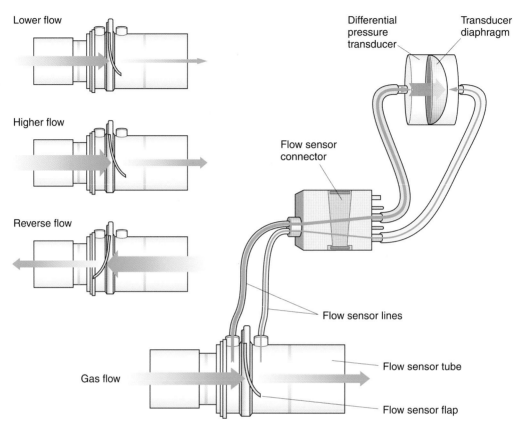

Figure 7-7 ▪ Variable orifice respirometer. (Reproduced with permission from Morgan GE, Mikhail MS, Murray MJ. *Clinical Anesthesiology*. 4th ed. New York, NY: McGraw-Hill; 2006. Figure 4-24C.)

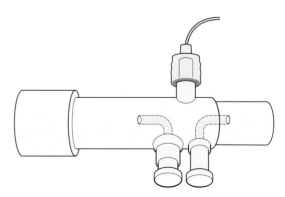

Figure 7-8 ▪ Fixed-orifice respirometer, as found in the Datex-Ohmeda D-Lite. (Reproduced with permission from Morgan GE, Mikhail MS, Murray MJ. *Clinical Anesthesiology*. 4th ed. New York, NY: McGraw-Hill; 2006. Figure 4-24D.)

a feedback loop can occur to correct for any changes in TV caused by changes in FGF (FGF compensation).

Airway Pressure Gauge

Somewhere in the circle is a monitor for airway pressure. The pressure monitoring system of a modern anesthesia machine measures peak airway pressure and subatmospheric pressure. Peak airway pressure measurements can be further divided into low peak airway pressure, sustained increased airway pressure, and high peak airway pressure. Alarms that are elicited by these measurements are important in proper patient monitoring; for instance, low peak airway pressure can be caused by a disconnect or overly low FGF. The limits for each of these parameters can be set by the operator or left to the default settings. The alarms are there for a purpose; they are not there to be ignored. If an alarm goes off, find out why. An airline pilot wouldn't keep hitting "silence alarms" in midflight without seeing what was going on.

Pressure Alarms

Built into the circle circuit at some place (the site varies from machine to machine) is a device that alarms based on certain parameters, such as low peak airway pressure, high peak airway pressure, sustained airway pressure, and subatmospheric pressure.

A low-pressure alarm is a type of fail-safe. It exists to tell us if there is a disconnect. In short, if the system does not detect a peak airway pressure above a certain amount over a certain time period, an alarm sounds to alert the user that there *may* be a disconnect. It is not a foolproof system. So how does it work?

If you look at your alarm settings, there will be one for minimum peak pressure, or *threshold* pressure. This is the minimum pressure reading that the alarm device will accept as being a breath. There must be at least one breath of a size or pressure that reaches the threshold value over a time span of 15 seconds. If there is no such breath over that time span, the alarm sounds.

There can be many causes of the low-pressure alarm to be set off. Low TVs, an endotracheal cuff leak, a circuit leak, and so forth are just some examples in addition to an actual disconnect or catastrophic leak. The low-pressure alarm is imprecise in telling you *what is wrong*, but its purpose is to tell you that *something is wrong*. It is up to you to troubleshoot the cause of the alarm using your clinical knowledge and experience.

The same pressure sensor will tell us if there is a high peak airway pressure; this is a value that may be set automatically by the machine or something that the operator sets. At any rate, you should be keenly aware of its setting.

Much harm can come from inadvertently high airway pressures, and peak airway pressures themselves can be an important diagnostic tool.

Likewise, sustained pressures and subatmospheric pressures can have a myriad of causes, which can be attributable to patient causes or machine causes.

The position in the circle circuit of airway pressure monitors vary from model to model of anesthesia machine. Most machines use electronic measuring sensors to sense airway pressure, but most modern machines have an analog "dial" type gauge in addition to digital screen readouts. The dial analog gauge is there as a backup in case the screen or the whole electrical system dies.

Many anesthesia machines now have software that allows flow volume loops to be generated based on the readings of the TVs and pressure changes during the respiratory cycle in real time. The loops are accessed via the menu of the machine's screen.

Positive End-Expiratory Pressure Valve

Although thought of predominately when discussing ventilators, the positive end-expiratory pressure (PEEP)–generating capability of anesthesia machines is found in the circuit, not the ventilator. PEEP generation involves adding resistance to expiration, usually through spring pressure on an expiratory unidirectional valve. PEEP valves are found somewhere along the expiratory portion of the circle circuit.

In the past, this was done by directly adjusting a knob coming out of the clear dome of the expiratory unidirectional valve, changing tension on a spring inside the apparatus (similar to a PEEP valve on a bag ventilator mask). Adjusting PEEP by the markings along this device was crude, and delivered PEEP versus dialed-in PEEP would likely differ. An even older PEEP device was an HME-type insert fitted between the expiratory limb and the expiratory limb port. The device had a ball bearing in it that provided gravity-induced resistance to exhalation. This PEEP valve had to be lined up perpendicular to the floor to work properly. They were not adjustable (or reusable); if you wanted to go from 5 cm H_2O to 10 cm H_2O, you had to use a different valve with a heavier ball bearing. If they were installed upside down, the circuit would be blocked totally (Figure 7-9).

Current anesthesia machines have PEEP valves that are electrically controlled that can precisely deliver whatever amount of PEEP is dialed into the ventilator controls. With electrically controlled PEEP valves, PEEP returns to zero when the machine is switched from ventilator to bag mode. With the older types mentioned, resistance to exhalation stayed the same when switching from ventilator to bag mode.

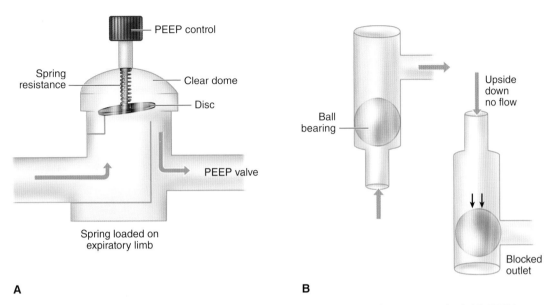

Figure 7-9 ▪ Spring-loaded positive end-expiratory pressure (PEEP) valve on the expiratory limb (**A**); PEEP insert at the expiratory limb (**B**). Note that if this PEEP valve was place upside down, the ball would block flow.

Filters

Filters are used to protect the patient from contamination from the machine and to protect the machine from contamination from the patient. Filters can be part of a new circle circuit right out of the bag or can be a separate component. For a long time, it was believed that contamination of a patient from an anesthesia machine was highly unlikely because of the high oxygen concentration found inside an anesthesia machine, the relative dryness inside a machine, and the highly alkaline environment in carbon dioxide absorbers. However, multiple case reports and studies have shown that bacterial and viral pathogens can be found inside anesthesia machines. *Mycobacterium tuberculosis* has been shown to be able to survive alkaline exposure from anesthesia machine carbon dioxide absorbers.

Mandatory use of filters is a controversial issue because of concerns over cost; effectiveness; increased resistance to breathing (especially in pediatric patients); and potential blockage of the filters, rendering ventilation impossible. The American Society of Anesthesiologists only recommends the use of antibacterial filters in patients with active tuberculosis.

The most effective filters for anesthesia machine use are those that are mechanical as opposed to electrostatic. Mechanical filters are made of pleated hydrophobic material that traps particles more effectively in moist conditions than electrostatic ones.

Table 7-1 PARTS OF A CIRCLE CIRCUIT	
Fresh gas inlet	Unidirectional valves
Inspiratory and expiratory ports	Circuit tubing
Y piece	Elbow
APL valve	Reservoir bag
Selector switch	Respirometer
Airway pressure gauge and alarm	PEEP valve
Filters	Carbon dioxide absorber

APL, adjustable pressure-limiting; PEEP, positive end-expiratory pressure.

Another controversial topic is the use of pleated hydrophobic filters in order to *reuse* a disposable circle circuit. Ideally, all that would be changed between patients would be a filter situated at the Y piece. Because it is at the Y piece, one filter would protect both the patient and the machine. Of course, the filter does not address any potential contamination on the *outside* of a reused circuit, along the tubing, the reservoir bag, and so on.

Carbon Dioxide Absorber

The carbon dioxide absorber is discussed in a separate chapter. It is placed *downstream* of the APL valve, so excess volume is released *upstream*. This way the absorbent isn't wasted on gas that is to be vented out anyway.

The parts of a circle circuit are summarized in Table 7-1.

ADVANTAGES OF THE CIRCLE CIRCUIT

Familiarity

Probably the main advantage of a circle circuit is that it is the most familiar type of circuit. Every anesthesiologist and anesthetist is comfortable in its use. In fact, it is probably the only circuit most of us have ever used with the exception of a Bain circuit.

Inhalational Agent Reuse

When the inhalational agent is at a level that is desired, FGF can be reduced because there is *rebreathing*. The inhalational agent that the patient exhales goes back around the circle and is reused, not counting what is lost to the scavenger system. The same goes for oxygen and nitrous oxide. This significantly reduces the cost of delivering an anesthetic because not as much inhalational agent is used than would be with, for example, a Bain circuit (where there is no rebreathing). There is also less pollution of the atmosphere (or the room if your scavenger is malfunctioning) because less agent is used.

Heat Loss Reduction

Studies confirm there is less heat loss with reduced flow rates that are only possible with a circle system. But don't think that using low flows will warm your patient efficiently. There is less humidity loss when using a circle system as well.

Mechanical Ventilation

The circle circuit is the only type of anesthesia circuit that can be used with mechanical ventilation, namely, the anesthesia machine ventilator.

DISADVANTAGES OF THE CIRCLE CIRCUIT

Complexity

You need an anesthesia machine to use a circle circuit, unlike a Bain circuit, for example. Also, there are many pieces to a circle circuit, which means there are more chances of a disconnect.

Increased Work of Breathing

There is resistance to breathing with a circle circuit. However, it is small and not really clinically significant even for infants. Dead space, as mentioned before, is more of a problem for infants than adults when a circle circuit is used.

HAZARDS OF THE CIRCLE CIRCUIT

Disconnects

There are several places that can become disconnected, for instance, the inspiratory and expiratory ports, Y piece and elbow, gas monitor sampling line, and reservoir bag.

Leaks

In our terminology, a disconnect is a *big* leak. Smaller leaks that do not cause a failure of ability to deliver positive-pressure ventilation can also occur, such as if the tubing is not securely pushed into the machine ports or if the plastic inspiratory and expiratory ports with an adjustable collar become loose, small to large holes in the corrugated tubing that may be difficult to find, and so forth (Figure 7-10).

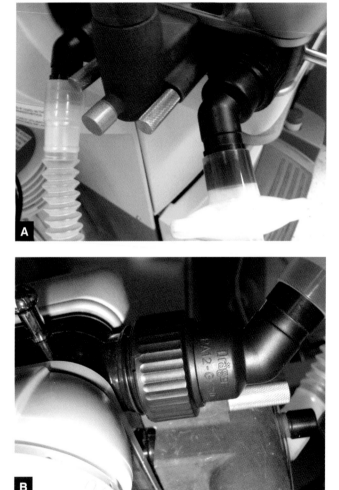

Figure 7-10 ▪ (**A**) and (**B**) Draeger Apollo inspiratory and expiratory limbs are adjustable, allowing one to change angle of the elbow bend by loosening black collars; if collars work loose or are not retightened after adjustment, a leak will occur.

Barotrauma

If the APL valve is closed enough, volume and pressure buildup can cause barotrauma. Looking back to see the reservoir bag the size of a basketball because you didn't open the APL valve all the way before you started taping in the endotracheal tube is a frightening event.

Rebreathing of Carbon Dioxide

One cause of carbon dioxide rebreathing is, of course, if the absorbent granules of the absorber need to be changed. This is mentioned in Chapter 9. Another cause of carbon dioxide rebreathing is an incompetent unidirectional valve, either inspiratory or expiratory.

Heat, Carbon Monoxide, and Compound A

These are discussed in Chapter 9 concerning the carbon dioxide absorber, but we include these as potential hazards because the absorber is an integral part of the circle system.

COAXIAL CIRCLE CIRCUIT

A coaxial circle is a type where, at first glance, there appears to be only one tube. However, if you look again, you will see a smaller tube *inside* the bigger tube. The external tube is clear and corrugated, and the internal tube is colored blue, green, or whatever so it is visible. The internal tubing is the inspiratory limb, and the external tubing is the expiratory limb. At the end that attaches to the machine, both limbs separate so you can attach them to the machine ports. The distal portion ends with an elbow similar to a regular circle (Figure 7-11).

A coaxial circuit cuts down on the "spaghetti" factor. Some believe that the inspiratory fresh gas is warmed by the surrounding expired gas because the inspiratory limb is within the expiratory limb. They are lighter in weight than a standard circle, so there is less pull on the endotracheal tube, facemask, or supraglottic device.

If, however, there is a kink in the inspiratory portion for any reason, it can be hard to detect. If the inspiratory limb is broken inside the expiratory limb, the circuit will still function, but dead space is increased because that portion distal to the break will functionally become a Y piece.

A FEW WORDS ABOUT NOMENCLATURE

You may have heard the phrases *semi-open, semi-closed*, and *closed circuit anesthesia*. What exactly do those terms mean?

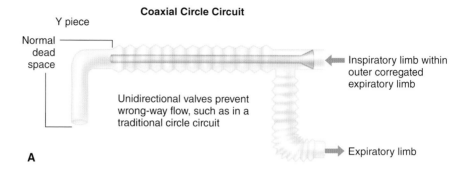

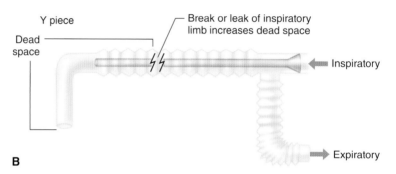

Figure 7-11 ▪ (**A**) Coaxial circle circuit. (**B**) Note that if a break or leak in inspiratory limb occurs, the space distal to leak becomes dead space.

These terms do not refer to a different kind of anesthesia circuit. It all has to do with how you are using a circle circuit. These terms have to do with the comparison of FGF and minute ventilation. They also have to do with the degree of rebreathing that is happening at a certain time. During an anesthetic, you may use each of these techniques.

For instance, at induction, most clinicians use high FGFs. This is an example of a semi-open circuit. If the FGF is greater than the minute ventilation, there is no net rebreathing. During maintenance of anesthesia, many people decrease the FGF. If the FGF is less than the minute ventilation, there is net rebreathing, and it is called semi-closed circuit anesthesia. The amount of rebreathing that occurs varies with what the FGF is. However, there is still some volume that goes to the scavenger system.

Some providers may even decrease FGF down to a point at which the FGF is equal to the metabolic requirements of oxygen, which is also called the patient uptake of oxygen. This is an example of closed circuit anesthesia.

Table 7-2	**COMPARISON OF SEMI-OPEN, SEMI-CLOSED, AND CLOSED CIRCUIT ANESTHESIA**
Semi-open	No net rebreathing; FGF > MV
Semi-closed	Some rebreathing occurs; MV > FGF > metabolic oxygen requirement
Closed	FGF = metabolic oxygen requirement

FGF, fresh gas flow; MV, minute ventilation.

There is complete rebreathing, so nothing (or virtually nothing) goes to the scavenger system.

Table 7-2 compares semi-open, semi-closed, and closed circuit anesthesia.

CONCLUSION

We hope you have enjoyed your journey around a circle anesthesia circuit. If things are not clear, hop on for another ride. The scenery will become more familiar.

ANESTHESIA MACHINE VENTILATORS | 8

Some anesthesia machine ventilators are visible, but others are inside the machine. You may think the ventilator is the "business end" of the machine, and in some ways you are correct. Use and manipulation of a ventilator are parts of acute care at its most acute—delivering oxygen to a patient that will cause the least amount of harm and the greatest amount of good. We will not discuss the physiology of ventilators in this chapter; that can be found in texts that do an infinitely better job of covering that topic. What we will discuss in this chapter is simply the mechanics of anesthesia machine ventilators.

There are a few different ways to ventilate a patient using an anesthesia machine. One is to use the mechanical ventilator that is built into the machine. Another way is to manually ventilate the patient with the reservoir bag ("bagging the patient"). Another method is jet ventilation using the machine's oxygen supply. Finally, the patient can breathe spontaneously while attached to the anesthesia machine. Each one of these methods has its place in anesthetic management.

Modern anesthesia machines are able to ventilate patients who would have been difficult to ventilate 20 years ago. Improvements in accuracy and power allow us to ventilate patients with stiff lungs that we could not have in the past. Back then an intensive care unit type ventilator may have been brought into the operating room (OR) simply to adequately ventilate such patients. In addition, with increases in accuracy and pressure monitoring and control, we are able to ventilate neonates and infants with a standard anesthesia machine ventilator now that would have been difficult in the past. Special smaller bellows were available for pediatric cases, and clinicians had to remove the standard size bellows and replace them with the smaller type for patients weighing less than around 10 kg.

There are two main types of anesthesia ventilators: bellows type and piston type. We will discuss each one in depth. Keep in mind, however, that machines can also be classified by what power source each one uses (purely pneumatic, pneumatic and electrical, or purely electrical). Although it is important to know how your anesthesia ventilator is powered, we prefer to classify them as to their mechanism of action.

A third type of anesthesia ventilator is the servo type. Formerly made by Siemens, they are now produced and marketed by Maquet. Those clinicians with experience in critical care may be familiar with the servo ventilator. These ventilators were modified to deliver volatile agents, and some even had rebreathing capability from an attached carbon dioxide absorber. Because of a servomechanism and its negative feedback, these ventilators were able to deliver tidal volumes (TVs) much more precisely than bellows-type anesthesia ventilators in the past, especially when dealing with the small TVs of neonates. Thus, the "servo" part of its name referred to its manner of ensuring proper TV delivery instead of how the ventilator itself worked. The means of delivering anesthetic agent is by an injection system into the fresh gas flow (FGF) instead of a traditional flow-over vaporizer. Nowadays, control of TV in modern anesthesia machines, whether bellows or piston type, has improved to the point where it is not difficult to ventilate neonates with a standard anesthesia machine.

BELLOWS VENTILATOR

The bellows-type ventilator may be the only type of anesthesia ventilator that many clinicians have ever used. Until the past decade, they were just about the only type available. Despite inroads made by the piston ventilator, bellows ventilators are ubiquitous, and generations of anesthesiologists and anesthetists have trained on them and use them tens of thousands of times each day.

The classification of bellows ventilators is as follows: pneumatically driven, double circuit, electronically controlled, ascending (or descending) bellows, time cycled, and TV preset. Similar to the classification of vaporizers, we will discuss each part of the description.

Pneumatically Driven

Exactly what makes the bellows move up and down? To the eye, there does not appear to be any mechanism that physically causes the bellows to move during a ventilatory cycle. Did you ever wonder why the bellows are in that clear plastic terrarium-like dome?

The reason is that on inspiration, that clear, airtight dome is pressurized with a gas that pushes the bellows down (or up in a descending bellows; more on that later). The gas is called the *driving gas*, and it is either oxygen or an oxygen and air mixture, depending on the type and brand of anesthesia machine. That is why the bellows ventilator is called *pneumatically driven*.

At the onset of inspiration, a valve opens, and the driving gas comes into the dome. The amount of driving gas needed per breath is approximately the same volume as the TV you have chosen to deliver. It is not exactly the same because there are other factors that are involved such as FGF, but for our purposes, we will say that the volume of pressurized driving gas is about the same as TV. This driving gas pushes the bellows, causing the volume of gas *inside* the bellows to enter the patient. At the end of inspiration, the valve letting the driving gas into the clear dome closes, and another valve opens that allows the driving gas to escape the clear dome. The bellows reexpand with the patient's passive exhalation because of the compliance of the chest wall. Then the cycle begins again (Figure 8-1).

As you can imagine, there is an incredible amount of driving gas used during an anesthetic. It is not recycled. After each breath, the driving gas is vented into the room. If you are using a cylinder source of oxygen, you will go through oxygen tanks relatively quickly. If the machine is the kind that uses an air–oxygen mix, air cylinders are not needed. The machine entrains air from an orifice in the back of the machine by the Venturi effect.

Because the driving gas is only oxygen or a mixture of oxygen and air, there is no pollution of the room with anesthetic agents. Remember, it is the

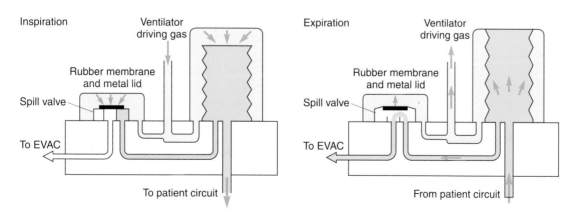

Figure 8-1 ▪ Schematic of a bellows ventilator. (Reproduced with permission from Morgan GE, Mikhail MS, Murray MJ. *Clinical Anesthesiology.* 2nd ed. New York, NY: McGraw-Hill; 2002. Figure 4-29.)

gas inside the bellows that goes into the patient and has anesthetic in it. The driving gas and the gas inside the bellows do not mix at all. (Actually they can mix, but we will talk about that later in the section Disadvantages and Hazards of Bellows Ventilators.)

Double Circuit

What this means is that there are two compartments of gas involved in a bellows-type anesthesia machine—the gas that is inside the bellows and the gas that is outside the bellows. As explained earlier, the gas outside the bellows is the driving gas that causes the bellows to move, and the gas inside the bellows is what goes into the patient. Under normal conditions, they never intermingle.

Electronically Controlled

Even though the bellows are pneumatically driven, the whole cycle relies on electricity to power the driving gas valves and to control the timing and volume of ventilation.

Ascending or Descending Bellows

By convention, bellows are named for what they do on expiration. They either go up or down. The only bellows ventilators you have ever used more than likely are the ascending type. Descending bellows fell out of favor in the late 1970s and early 1980s. They were believed to be a safety hazard.

Ascending bellows are anchored to the bottom of the clear dome. They move down on inspiration and fill back up again on expiration. Descending bellows, as you can guess, do the opposite of ascending bellows. They are anchored to the top of the clear dome. Imagine a bat hanging upside down. They move up on inspiration and move down as they reexpand. Ascending bellows have a small amount of intrinsic positive end-expiratory pressure (PEEP) as a result of the weight of the bellows being pushed back up on exhalation, somewhere around 1 to 2 cm H_2O.

If there is a disconnect, what happens to *ascending* bellows? They collapse because of loss of pressure inside them and gravity. The low-pressure alarm goes off, and you see the collapsed bellows. This has been a tremendous visual aid over the years, especially in the days before routine capnography. Experienced clinicians rely on visual cues from the ascending bellows a great deal. Not only do ascending bellows give a visual indication of a disconnect, but they also give a visual cue of a leak. If there is a leak in the circuit, the bellows will not rise all the way to the top of the clear dome after each breath. In addition, ascending bellows give the clinician a visual cue of when the patient "breathes through" the ventilator, initiating spontaneous respirations are returning.

The main problem with *descending* bellows is what happens during a disconnect. Because of gravity, the descending bellows elongate when there is a loss of pressure and volume. They look like they are full, but actually the opposite is occurring. Remember, when the ascending bellows lose volume and pressure, they collapse, leaving an empty clear dome, which is a good visual alarm to an anesthetist that something is wrong.

In addition to *not* giving you a visual clue of a disconnect, a descending bellows disconnect might not cause enough of a pressure change to sound the low-pressure alarm.

However, one company, Datascope/Anestar, has produced a machine with descending bellows in the 2000s. The company says the problem of undetected disconnect with a descending bellows is not a factor now because the apnea alarm comes from the capnograph, not the machine itself.

Nevertheless, the two main anesthesia machine companies, Datex-Ohmeda and Draeger, produce ascending bellows machines.

Time Cycled

We control by electric means the number of breaths per minute.

Tidal Volume Preset

We control by electrical means the TV that will be delivered to a patient. Modern bellows machines can also use pressure control, where the peak airway pressure the operator wishes to administer is set and the TV is a result of that pressure.

Disadvantages and Hazards of Bellows Ventilators

Tidal Volume Accuracy

As stated, inspiration is initiated because the driving gas enters the clear dome and pressurizes it, and as more driving gas enters, the bellows are pushed down to deliver the set TV to the patient. There is more variability in each breath potentially because of changes in patient lung compliance and airway resistance. The driving gas is compressible, so as an example, the same amount of driving gas that pushed the bellows down to deliver 700 cc TV on one breath and one level of lung compliance and airway resistance may not make the bellows move the same amount on the next breath if compliance and resistance vary from one breath to another. It is the compressibility of the driving gas that is the main problem with TV accuracy with a bellows ventilator.

Use of Oxygen as Driving Gas

As discussed earlier, bellows ventilators use a lot of oxygen. The amount will be around what your minute ventilation is. It is not recyclable. Even with some machine types that use oxygen and entrained room air, quite a bit of oxygen is used. This can be problematic if you are in an anesthetizing location that does not have a wall source for oxygen. The driving gas for the ventilator would have to come from your oxygen cylinders.

Let us go through an example. You are anesthetizing in a location that has no wall or pipeline source of oxygen. You are delivering a TV of 700 cc at a rate of 10 breaths/min. The minute volume therefore is 7 L/min. So you are using approximately 7 L/min just to operate the bellows. After 1 hour of anesthesia, your utilization of oxygen just to drive the bellows is

$$7 \text{ L/minute} \times 60 \text{ minutes} = 420 \text{ L}$$

Your oxygen cylinder has 660 L of oxygen in it.

$$420 \text{ L} \div 660 \text{ L} = 64\%$$

So you have used two thirds of your E-cylinder of oxygen simply to drive the bellows! This leaves you with 240 L to oxygenate the patient, which averages out to 4 L/min to use for patient oxygenation. It is easy to run low flows during the maintenance of an anesthetic, but most clinicians use higher flows for induction and emergence and to rapidly change inhalational concentration. Don't forget the oxygen flush button either!

What it boils down to is that you would have to change out cylinders every hour or so. That would be not only a hassle to change them so frequently and lug that many tanks to your location but also potentially dangerous for the patient. Who is going to change the tank? Can they do it quickly? If you change the tank, who will watch the patient while you are behind the machine?

Leaks

As mentioned previously, pediatric-sized bellows were available in the past before the accuracy of bellows ventilators improved. The bellows were easily changed out in only a couple of minutes. However, each time the bellows were changed, it introduced a chance for leaks to happen if the bellows assembly was not exactly fitted properly onto the ventilator. In those days, the bellows attachment was a commonplace to find circuit leaks. Fortunately, we do not have to change bellows anymore. The same bellows ventilator can safely and accurately ventilate an adult or an infant.

Be on guard for bellows assembly leaks if any maintenance was recently done on your machine. The black plastic bellows need to be replaced every once in a while, so improper reassembly can result in a leak.

Another type of leak reported with bellows is when there is a hole in the bellows themselves. Remember we said the bellows assembly is a "double circuit" with one volume of gas inside the bellows that goes into the patient and a separate volume inside the dome assembly that is our driving gas. These two volumes of gas are separate and never intermingle.

With a hole in the bellows, though, the two different volumes of gas can mix. The pressure in the clear dome is around 50 psig when it is pressurized and the bellows are pushed down. That high pressure can potentially be transmitted through the hole in the bellows and cause barotrauma to the patient.

In addition, the fraction of inspired oxygen (FiO_2) can change because of a hole in the bellows. The 100% oxygen that is the driving gas in an Ohmeda machine or the oxygen–air mixture in a Draeger bellows machine can either dilute or enrich your FiO_2, depending on the circumstance if a hole in the bellows allows the two sections of gas to mix.

Barotrauma

In addition to high pressure being transmitted through the bellows from the driving gas in case of a bellows hole, barotrauma can also occur from using the oxygen flush button during inspiration.

| PISTON DRIVE

The piston drive ventilator is relatively simpler than the bellows. It may seem a bit more mysterious to you because it is sometimes hidden deep inside the anesthesia machine. See Figures 8-2 and 8-3 as examples of how to access the piston on a Draeger Apollo machine. The piston drive ventilator consists of a cylinder, about the size of a coffee can that contains a soft, flexible plastic insert reminiscent of a flower pot. There is a piston at one end of the cylinder. A motor actuates on inspiration to push the piston to whatever degree it takes to deliver the set TV. The piston pushes the gas volume of the flexible insert into the patient circuit (Figures 8-4 and 8-5).

The housing of the piston is heated. It is not heated to warm inspired gases for the patient. The reason the housing is heated is to prevent moisture condensation because there are many electronic parts in the housing.

There are no visual cues with a piston drive for things such as spontaneous respirations. A disconnect, however, will cause the reservoir bag to empty.

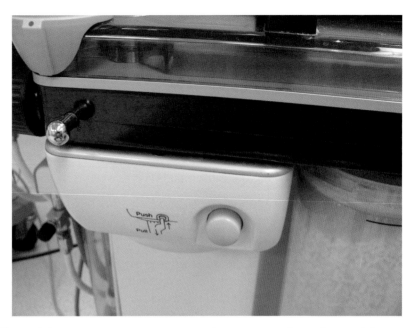

Figure 8-2 ▪ Access button to the inside of a Draeger Apollo machine and the piston drive ventilator.

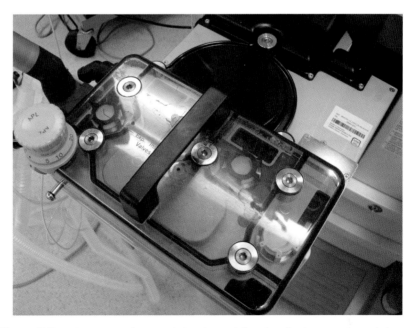

Figure 8-3 ▪ Access panel opened showing unidirectional valves on top and the top of piston drive (black circular lid) behind.

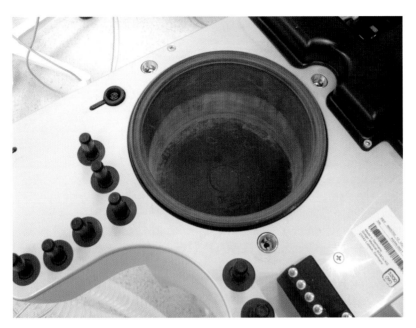

Figure 8-4 ▪ Deformable liner of a piston drive exposed; a gasket-like rim of liner forms an airtight seal with the top panel, which has been removed.

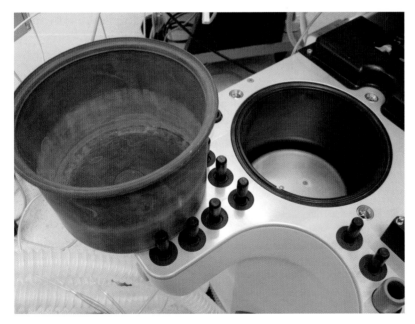

Figure 8-5 ▪ With the liner of the piston drive removed, the piston head is seen in the cylinder.

(The reservoir bag is a part of the ventilator circuit with a piston drive; more on this later.)

There is less influence of patient lung compliance on a piston drive compared with a bellows ventilator. The piston moves the required distance in it cylinder to deliver the set TV, back and forth, until you change the settings or until the circuit reaches your high value for peak airway pressure. There is no intrinsic PEEP in the piston ventilator.

There is no need for a driving gas in piston ventilators. They are totally electrically driven and powered. Therefore, piston ventilators would be the better choice when oxygen supply is limited.

Disadvantages

There really are no serious disadvantages to a piston drive ventilator. They are quiet and hidden, which may be strange to an older generation of anesthetists who were used to hearing and seeing the bellows work. Some piston machines have an artificial sound that can be turned on. As mentioned, there are no visual cues for spontaneous breathing. Disconnects cause the reservoir bag to empty as a visual sign (Table 8-1).

Table 8-1 **COMPARISON BETWEEN BELLOWS VERSUS PISTON VENTILATORS**		
	Bellows	Piston
Power source	Electric	Electric
Driving mechanism	Pneumatic	Mechanical piston
Driving gas needed	Yes	No
FGF compensatory mechanism	FGF compensation	FGF decoupling
Need to change components for pediatric or neonatal patients	Yes (older models) No (modern models)	No
Volume control mode	Yes	Yes
Pressure-controlled mode	Yes (modern models)	Yes
Visual cue of disconnect	Yes	No
Pressure support	Yes (modern models)	Yes
Is reservoir bag part of circuit?	No	Yes

FGF, fresh gas flow.

FRESH GAS FLOW COMPENSATION AND DECOUPLING

This is an important topic, but it may be confusing to you at first. If you don't understand after the first time you read this, take a deep breath and read it again. It should start to make sense. Also, ask an older clinician to explain the influence that FGF used to have on TVs with older machines.

In the past, up until the 2000s, FGF influenced TV on anesthesia machine ventilators. Delivered TV was the sum of the set TV plus FGF. When using the anesthesia machine ventilator, each time you changed your FGF, your TV you were running changed: increased FGF would increase TV, and decreased FGF would decrease TV. So the operator had to adjust their TV each time the FGF was changed to keep the TV where he or she wanted it. This may sound like a big chore to you, but we older clinicians were used to it, and there wasn't any other way to deal with it anyway.

Modern machines now automatically keep the TV that is set from being influenced by changes in FGF. There are two methods in which this occurs. One is called *fresh gas flow compensation*, and the other is called *fresh gas flow decoupling*. We will, of course, discuss each one.

Fresh Gas Flow Compensation

This may be the easier of the two to understand. There are volume sensors in the circle circuit that compare the set TV to the delivered and returned TV. When FGF is changed, TV *is initially influenced*, but these feedback loops tell the ventilator to adjust how much the bellows is depressed (by changing the volume of driving gas that enters the bellows chamber, remember?). So within 3 or 4 breaths, the TV has returned to what you have dialed in. This system is common in Datex-Ohmeda machines.

Fresh Gas Flow Decoupling

This is the type of system commonly found on piston drive machines, but it can also be found on some bellows-type ventilators. When the piston starts to move at the initiation of inspiration, the FGF is *diverted* through a valve to the reservoir bag. On exhalation, the valve changes again and allows the piston cylinder to be refilled by the FGF coming from not only the pneumatic part of the machine but also the reservoir bag. If you notice on a piston-type machine, the bag moves in and out during the ventilator cycle, almost like the patient is breathing spontaneously. But on further inspection, the movements are the opposite of what you see in spontaneous ventilation. The bag expands slightly on inspiration (because the FGF is being *diverted* into it) and gets slightly smaller on expiration (because the piston cylinder is refilling with some of the reservoir bag contents).

Therefore, the FGF is *decoupled* from the ventilator during the cycle. Actually, the authors prefer to call it *fresh gas flow diverting* because diverting seems easier to understand than decoupling.

With fresh gas decoupling, the oxygen flush button is *decoupled* from the piston on inspiration, so if the button is pressed during inspiration, there will be no effect on circuit pressure or volume.

CONCLUSION

We certainly hope you have a better understanding of anesthesia ventilators. Like we mentioned at the beginning of this chapter, this was about the nuts and bolts of how the machine ventilator works. You will need to consult other texts to obtain an understanding about the physiology of mechanical ventilation.

CARBON DIOXIDE ABSORBER 9

KEYWORDS

- CO_2 absorption
- carbon dioxide absorption
- efficiency
- Compound A
- carbon monoxide

The hallmark of a circle anesthesia circuit is *rebreathing*. Of course, a circle circuit is not a true circle, but it is a continuous path recycling the gases and anesthetic vapors you have chosen by your flowmeters and vaporizers. The only things not part of the recycling process are what comes in from the fresh gas inlet and what goes out to the scavenger system. *How much* is recycled depends on your fresh gas flow (FGF; described in more detail in another section).

The three important things in a circle system are the two unidirectional valves (one inspiratory, one expiratory) and the carbon dioxide absorber. At low or normal FGF rates, lack of a means to get rid of CO_2 would quickly lead to rebreathing and hypercarbia, just like breathing into a paper bag. This chapter will describe how the carbon dioxide absorption system in an anesthesia machine works.

A BRIEF HISTORY

Similar to many technical innovations, carbon dioxide absorption capability is a result of exploration and military advances. In this case, mining, underwater exploration, and submarine development were the catalysts for developing a reliable way to "scrub" CO_2 out of a closed environment. Various means of rebreathing have been described since the 1700s, and by the late 19th century, soda lime was in use as an absorbent. The Davis Escape Set was invented and produced at the turn of the 20th century as a means of rescue from disabled submarines. It was a self-contained vest and mask system containing oxygen and barium hydroxide. By 1912, Draeger (yes, *that* Draeger) was mass producing rebreathers for German navy divers. In 1923, the pioneering anesthesiologist Dr. Ralph Waters incorporated a CO_2 absorption system into an anesthesia circuit, beginning the practice of low-flow anesthesia and reuse of agent with the patient rebreathing his own scrubbed exhalations. Since then, circle anesthesia systems and rebreathing have become the most commonly used means of delivery of inhalational anesthetics.

DESIGN

The typical anesthesia machine absorber is a clear plastic canister or collection of canisters of varying sizes but at least of the same volume as a patient's typical tidal volume. The canister is full of some type of alkaline absorbent granules. The canisters are incorporated into the ventilatory apparatus of the anesthesia machine between the expiratory and inspiratory limbs of a circle circuit. The setup is located as to be visible to the anesthesia provider because visual inspection of its status and operation is important. At expiration, that expired volume travels through the absorber canister and is exposed to the absorbent granules, where the CO_2 is converted to carbonic acid and then to carbonate, water, and heat. So, in actuality it is a simple conversion of a base to an acid.

In some designs, the expired gas enters the absorber canister from the top and travels to the bottom before being piped back up into the rest of the ventilatory apparatus. In other designs, the expired gas travels down the middle of the canister in a center tube and then flows upward through the granules (Figure 9-1). This means that in some designs, the purple, exhausted granules will be on the top of the canisters or at the bottom of the canister (Figures 9-2 and 9-3).

Canisters have built-in baffles to disperse the flow of gas throughout the absorbent granules to reduce channeling (discussed later). Canisters also often have spaces where granule dust and excess moisture can accumulate, to be emptied later.

On the Datex-Ohmeda ADU machine, the canisters are disposable and pop on and off a small platform that is self-sealing, allowing quick changes during an anesthetic without loss of fresh gas volume (Figure 9-4). These prefilled canisters are more expensive than bags of loose granules used to refill reusable canisters. Other, newer Datex-Ohmeda machines also have disposable canisters (Figure 9-5). Draeger also has disposable prefilled canisters that can be changed quite easily.

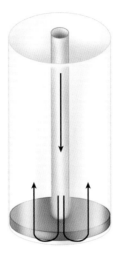

Figure 9-1 ▪ Schematic of Draeger design canister.

Newer designs of absorbers have smaller volumes in their canisters than in the past. This is done to force the user to change the granules more frequently because in a smaller canister, the granules become exhausted more quickly. Changing the granules more frequently decreases the incidence of granule desiccation and therefore decreases formation of carbon monoxide and Compound A.

ABSORBENTS

Traditionally, absorbent granules have been made from soda lime, a mixture of strong bases, such as sodium hydroxide, potassium hydroxide, and the weaker base calcium hydroxide. As it turns out, these strongly basic absorbent materials are more likely to produce carbon monoxide and Compound A when desiccated compared with absorbents made from weaker bases. Most types of granules now use a mixture containing more calcium hydroxide, with fewer amounts of the stronger bases. There are also preparations of absorbents that are proprietary mixtures (Draegersorb) and do not make clinically significant amounts of carbon monoxide and Compound A.

The shape and size of the absorbent are important. They are produced in either pellet- or gravel-shaped granules of a size that is a compromise between surface area and solidness. Smaller granules are more prone to being crushed into powder during handling, and larger granules would have less surface area.

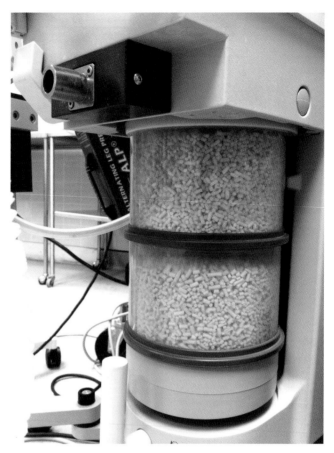

Figure 9-2 ▪ Datex-Ohmeda stacked canisters showing depleted (purple) granules on top; expired gas travels down through canisters and then back up to the circuit.

Silica is added to keep the granules from falling apart. This preserves the correct granule size, and it decreases absorbent dust, which would be toxic if inspired. The unit of measure of size is called "mesh," which reflects the number of holes in a screen per square inch; absorbent granules are between 4 and 8 mesh.

Absorbent granules contain a chemical indicator that changes color with changes in pH. As the beige or off white granules become exhausted of ability to absorb CO_2, they change to a light purple color because of the presence of the indicator ethyl violet. This is the reason that absorbers are made of clear plastic.

Soda lime neutralizes between 14 and 23 L of carbon dioxide for each 100 g of absorbent. The chemical reaction that occurs needs water to occur

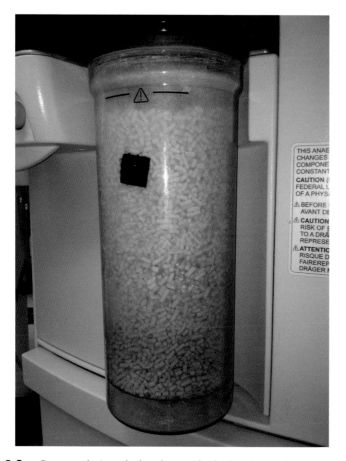

Figure 9-3 ▪ Draeger-designed absorber, with depleted (purple) granules at the bottom of the column. Expired gas travels down a center tube to the bottom of the canister and then upward. The empty space at bottom is where the baffle is that decreases channeling and where dust and moisture are trapped.

(to change carbon dioxide into carbonic acid), so absorbent is typically 155 to 20% water by content. The reaction is as follows for a generic absorbent that contains both sodium hydroxide and calcium hydroxide:

$$CO_2 + H_2O \rightarrow H_2CO_3 + H_2O + Heat$$
$$H_2CO_3 + 2NaOH \rightarrow Na_2CO_3 + 2H_2O + Heat$$
$$Na_2CO_3 + Ca(OH)_2 \rightarrow CaCO_3 + 2NaOH$$

Note that the end product is sodium hydroxide (lye). Any water that forms in an absorbent canister should be considered hazardous.

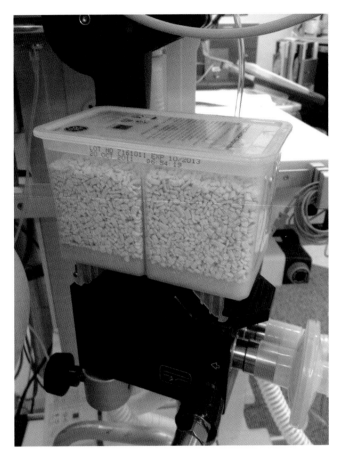

Figure 9-4 ▪ A Datex-Ohmeda ADU disposable absorber canister.

HAZARDS OF CARBON DIOXIDE ABSORBERS

There are several hazards and adverse outcomes that can occur because of an anesthesia machine's CO_2 absorbent system.

Leaks

The canisters themselves can be the site of leaks, usually very large leaks, because of improper placement of the canisters into the apparatus. The canisters have built-in gaskets that must be properly situated in order to be air tight, not only the canister-to-apparatus interface but also if canisters are stacked. Wayward granules, hanging cables, and so on can also be trapped between seals, causing a leak. One of the authors even once had an unintentional

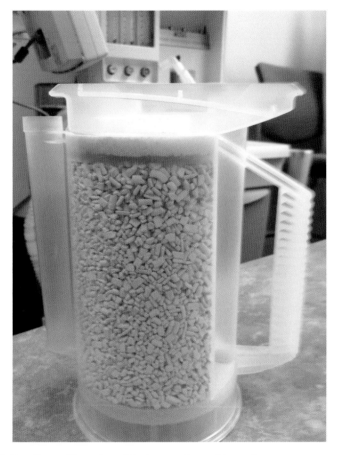

Figure 9-5 ▪ Datex-Ohmeda quick-change disposable canister.

sabotage of the absorber when a new anesthesia technician placed the wrong manufacturer's canisters on a machine while replacing the granules between cases, resulting in a catastrophic leak.

Compound A

Compound A is vinyl ether that is produced as a reaction between sevoflurane and the absorbent. It is important to remember that Compound A is *not* a metabolic byproduct of sevoflurane; its formation occurs outside the body in the absorbent canister itself. Compound A is nephrotoxic in rats. Multiple studies regarding its potential to be nephrotoxic in humans have been published, and readers are directed to those articles for more information.

The formation of Compound A involves many variables. Low FGFs are associated with Compound A formation. Compound A is produced in greater levels when absorbents containing sodium and potassium hydroxides are used. It is also seen in higher concentrations when the absorbent granules are desiccated and when the canister temperature is higher than normal. More Compound A is seen in longer anesthetics and anesthetics using higher concentrations of sevoflurane.

Carbon Monoxide

Carbon monoxide in clinically significant concentrations can be seen as a byproduct of the interaction of desiccated absorbents with desflurane and isoflurane. It is seen with sevoflurane only if the canister temperature becomes very high (e.g., 80°C, which can happen with sevoflurane; see later discussion). One study showed that carbon monoxide can be formed with sevoflurane and dry absorbent in canisters of normal temperature.

Incidents involving carbon monoxide formation in absorbents were initially reported as happening on Monday mornings with the first anesthetic that day. This scenario is explained by the machine being left on with gas flowing through the absorbent over the weekend, causing the granules to dry out. Little-used machines with dry granules have also been implicated in carbon monoxide formation.

Fire

Melting of plastic components and even flames have been reported when sevoflurane has been used in machines with dried-out absorbent granules. This was more common when barium hydroxide (baralyme) was still in use as an absorbent ingredient, but it has also been seen with other formulations of absorbent granules.

Dust and Moisture

Because absorbents are made from alkaline substances, they should be handled with care. Dust can irritate eyes and skin, and any water that collects in the canisters should be handled very carefully because of its strong base properties.

Channeling

Channeling occurs when the gas flow through the absorbent granules follows the path of least resistance, thereby exhausting the exposed granules in that path. The path is sometimes in the middle of the canister, with the purple

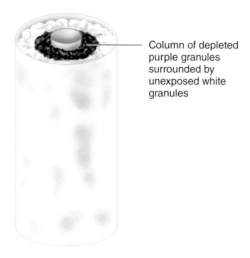

Column of depleted purple granules surrounded by unexposed white granules

Figure 9-6 ▪ Channeling.

granules hidden by little- or unexposed granules. Channeling causes inspired CO_2 to appear when the granules visible still appear good. Proper filling of canisters to eliminate less dense pockets of granules by tapping the canisters on the work area while filling them limits channeling (Figure 9-6).

CONCLUSION

This chapter has shown that something we almost always ignore is that the carbon dioxide absorbent system of the anesthesia machine is actually complex. Not only is it complex, but you should also see that the absorber is not a benign part of the machine. Harm can happen to a patient through several ways because of the absorber, so we should be familiar with how it works, the potential hazards, and how we can prevent those hazards from happening during anesthetic cases.

SCAVENGER SYSTEM | 10

Let's say you are performing an anesthetic. You have the fresh gas flow (FGF) at 2 L/min. We know that the FGF enters the circle circuit, joining the exhaled gas that will be rebreathed. But eventually, what happens to all the gas and vapor we control with our flowmeters and vaporizers? It has to go someplace. It has to leave the machine; otherwise, the machine would explode.

There is an exhaust for the machine. It is called the *scavenger system*. But it is more than merely the tail pipe for the anesthesia machine. It has a role in protecting you and the rest of the people in the OR. This assembly takes all the gas that leaves the machine and directs it out of the operating room (OR) so we are not exposed to the waste anesthetics. A properly adjusted scavenger system's output is the same as the FGF.

TYPES OF SYSTEMS

There are two main types of scavenger systems, classified by whether medical suction is used to evacuate the exhaust gas. An *active system* requires wall or pipeline suction to evacuate the waste gas. A *passive system* relies on the upstream flow of gas coming out of the machine to passively flow out of the system, similar to how water flows through and out of a garden hose (a garden hose doesn't need suction at the end of it to pull the water out of it).

Active System

As stated, an active system must be attached to some form of suction or evacuation unit, which would be the facility wall or pipeline suction. In most instances, there are separate plug-ins on the wall for scavenging suction and patient suction. Somewhere in the scavenger apparatus, there will be a means of adjusting the negative pressure from the wall, so the suction will not be too strong or too weak to be effective.

Active systems need some form of negative pressure relief to ensure the suction will not be so strong as to create a vacuum within the anesthesia machine itself. An active system also needs some type of positive pressure relief in case suction is not adequate or is disrupted so positive pressure will not build up in the anesthesia machine. In fact, one of the possible hazards of scavenger systems is barotrauma to the patient if the scavenger suction is not strong enough or is not working at all.

Passive System

A passive system is a low-pressure system that relies on the passive flow of gas out of the machine and is connected to some sort of egress out of the room so as to not pollute the OR (which is, remember, the whole purpose of the scavenger in the first place).

Unlike active systems, there is no risk of developing too much negative pressure, so a negative-pressure relief valve is not needed. However, there is the possibility of high pressure building up if the passive flow is impeded, so a high-pressure relief valve is necessary.

The exit of the waste gas from the anesthetizing location can be as simple as a hole in an outside wall to a ventilation duct with a fan to assist the gas out of the area.

INTERFACES

We have just discussed the two types of scavenger systems, active and passive. Now we need to talk about the two different types of *interfaces*. What is an interface? An interface classifies the scavenger system's relationship to its environment. A scavenger system can be *open* or *closed* to its environment.

An active system can either have an open or closed interface. A passive system can have only a closed interface. If you are confused, don't worry. All of this will be explained simply.

Open Interface

An open interface is a scavenger system that is actually open to the room environment (Figures 10-1 and 10-2). The scavenger itself will have holes or slits in the apparatus itself that allow protection of the patient to both positive and negative barotrauma. The scavenger will have what looks like a flowmeter

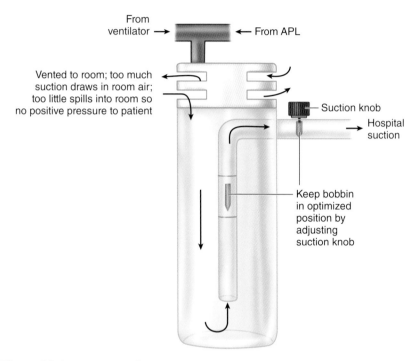

From ventilator →

← From APL

Vented to room; too much suction draws in room air; too little spills into room so no positive pressure to patient

Suction knob

Hospital suction

Keep bobbin in optimized position by adjusting suction knob

Figure 10-1 ▪ Open interface scavenger system. APL, adjustable pressure-limiting.

device as part of its construction with a bobbin inside. The goal is to keep the bobbin within the factory-set lines or zone by adjusting the strength of the wall suction. This allows for the proper amount of suction, individualized for each anesthetizing location. This is important because suction strength can vary from room to room or location to location. Remember in our discussion about active systems we said that such a system required a means of both negative pressure relief and positive pressure relief. In an open interface, this is achieved because of the open system itself. If suction is too strong, the unit will entrain room air to satisfy the suction power instead of sucking it out of the machine. If suction is too weak, the unit will let the excess volume vent into the room instead of causing increased pressure in the anesthesia machine and potential barotrauma to the patient (Figure 10-3).

All of this is done without moving parts or valves with springs that get old, rusty, and dust covered and that are prone to sticking. After all, when was the last time you checked the pressure relief valves on your scavenger system? Of course, no one ever does. That is the beauty of the open interface.

Okay, the open interface provides safety for the patient, but what about the safety of the anesthetist and anybody else in the room in the event that the suction to the scavenger is not strong enough or someone rolled a heavy

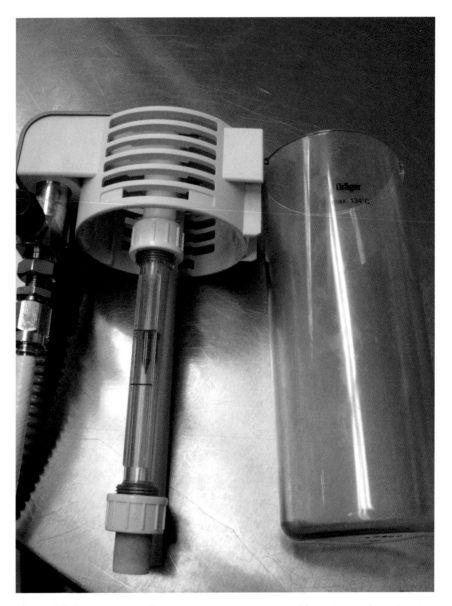

Figure 10-2 ■ Open interface scavenger system removed from the machine showing details.

object over the scavenger suction wall tubing? Well, there will be pollution of the room because the open interface will let the waste gas exit into the room. But remember the word "vigilance?" It is up to the operator of the anesthesia machine to ensure the scavenger is working. Any unexplained odor of inhalational agent needs to be investigated. The flowmeter bobbin of the

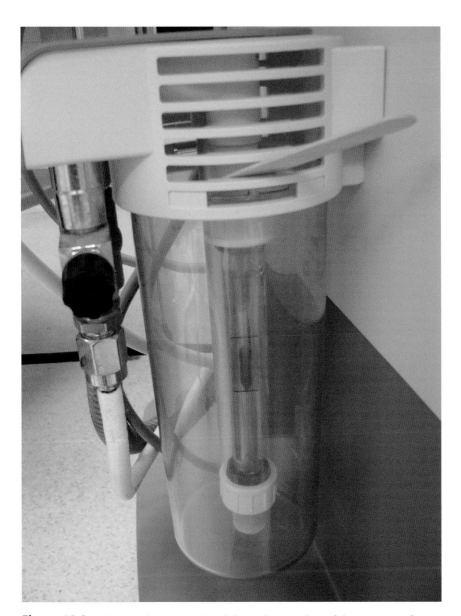

Figure 10-3 ▪ Tongue depressor placed through open slots of the open interface to show communication with room atmosphere.

open interface should be checked often to make sure it is floating where it is supposed to be.

An open interface needs active suction to function. If an open interface was part of a passive system, the waste gas would simply vent into the room through the holes or slits of the interface.

Most anesthesia machines have the scavenger situated so that it is easily visible from the operator's position. Unfortunately, not all are as user friendly. For example, on some Datex-Ohmeda machines, the scavenger or its flowmeter is on the back of the machine and not visible from the front at all.

Closed Interface

This type of interface is closed to room air. A closed interface can be part of either an active or passive system. It works with (active system) or without (passive system) suction. A passive closed interface is more or less a hose that connects to the anesthesia machine exhaust and is diverted out of the room. It needs a positive-pressure relief valve so pressure can be vented if there is an obstruction to flow of some kind downstream of the machine (Figure 10-4).

A closed interface unit for an active system is more complex. It is situated so as to be visible from the anesthetist's station at the front of the anesthesia machine. It consists of a connection to both the machine and the suction tubing, a knob to control the amount of suction, positive- and negative-pressure relief valves, and a reservoir bag.

The tubing that goes from the machine itself to the interface may be incorporated into the design of the anesthesia machine and not be visible. Or it may be situated on the outside of the machine. The kind that is on the outside of the machine may resemble the corrugated tubing of our anesthesia circle circuit, but for safety reasons, the scavenger system has been made with different sized connectors, so the misplacing of the patient circuit to the scavenger circuit is not possible. This tubing needs to be of a length so as not to drag along the floor, where it could become obstructed or damaged.

Another distinctive part of a closed interface for active suction is a reservoir bag. Again, to not risk being mistaken for the reservoir bag of the patient circuit, it is out of reach (but visible) and is usually colored differently and has different sized connectors than the patient reservoir bag.

The scavenger reservoir bag is something that needs to be inspected often to make sure it is working properly. The shape of the bag is a big deal when talking about closed interface scavengers. When the suction is adjusted, the shape of the reservoir bag changes. The goal is to keep the bag shaped somewhat like a football. If it is round like a basketball, there is not enough suction. If the bag is flat as a pancake, there is too much suction.

Closed interfaces have spring-loaded pressure relief valves. Negative-pressure valves are set at around -0.5 to -2 cm H_2O and positive-pressure relief valves are designed to vent at 5 cm H_2O. These valves can be overlooked easily when a machine is inspected. Dirt, dust, dried oil, and the like can cause them to stick.

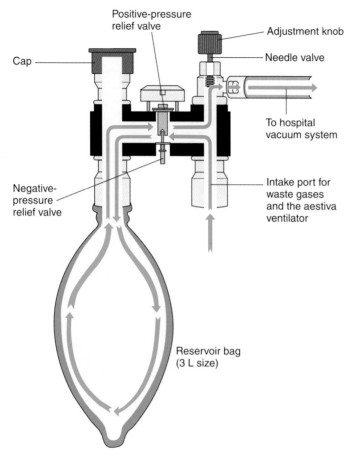

Positive-pressure
relief valve

Adjustment knob

Cap

Needle valve

To hospital
vacuum system

Negative-
pressure
relief valve

Intake port for
waste gases
and the aestiva
ventilator

Reservoir bag
(3 L size)

Figure 10-4 ▪ Closed interface scavenger system. (Reproduced with permission from Morgan GE, Mikhail MS, Murray MJ. *Clinical Anesthesiology.* 4th ed. New York, NY: McGraw-Hill; 2006. Figure 4-32C.)

HAZARDS OF SCAVENGER SYSTEMS

Occupational Exposure to Waste Anesthetic Gases and Vapors

This is a very old topic and one that has no real clear-cut answers. In the past, it was thought that chronic occupational exposure to waste anesthetic gases or vapors *might* cause cancer, hepatitis, miscarriages, birth defects, or decreased vigilance in OR personnel. This has never been shown conclusively to be true, and you can find multiple studies that will say yes or no to the question.

Of course, one cannot prospectively test chronic exposure of anesthetic gases and subsequent results on humans but merely collect data on humans who have had chronic workplace exposure. Studies on animals, however, have not shown conclusively any truth to the matter even with exposing laboratory animals to very high levels of waste gas, many times more than would be even in an OR that did not have a scavenger system.

Nevertheless, it is something that has not been proven, but people are still worried about it. The National Institute for Occupational Safety and Health (NIOSH) has recommendations about what levels of anesthetic agents are acceptable in the room air of an anesthetizing location. For nitrous oxide, the level should be less than 25 parts per million (ppm) and 2 ppm for the halogenated anesthetics. If nitrous oxide and a halogenated agent are used at the same time, the level acceptable for nitrous oxide is less than 25 and 0.5 ppm for the agent. Keep in mind that if you can detect anesthetic vapor by smell, the concentration is at least 30 ppm. Nitrous oxide has no odor.

Can inhaling waste anesthetic gases impede one's performance? Will it make you sleepy? This has also been studied a lot over the years. In concentrations less than the NIOSH recommendations, it is believed that there are no negative psychomotor effects associated with waste anesthetic gases.

The American Society of Anesthesiologists' Task Force on Waste Anesthetic Gases report states: "Studies have not shown an association between trace levels of waste anesthetic gases found in scavenged anesthetizing locations and adverse health effects to personnel." Nevertheless, their recommendation is: "Waste anesthetic gases should be scavenged."

Excess Positive Pressure

If the scavenger is not working properly or the tubing is kinked or obstructed somehow, positive pressure could build up and make its way to the patient circuit. With an open interface, the obstruction would have to be between the machine and the interface itself because an open interface can very easily vent excess pressure into the room. A closed interface system will have a positive-pressure relief valve that is designed to open at 5 cm H_2O of positive pressure within the scavenger. But there is a bit more risk that a closed interface would fail to vent excess pressure because the mechanical valves found on them can fail to work for various reasons, such as neglect in maintenance, dust buildup, and so forth.

Excess Negative Pressure

The suction applied to a scavenger system can be so strong that it can suck the gas out of the patient circuit and reservoir bag. If spontaneously breathing, the patient would generate negative pressure in his or her airway and potentially cause negative-pressure pulmonary edema. Even if the scavenger did not evacuate all the gas out of the circuit, the flow rate of a spontaneously breathing patient is much higher than the usual FGF of an anesthesia machine, so the patient would run out of gas (more importantly, oxygen) to inhale from the machine, causing hypoxia as well as the risk of pulmonary edema.

Open interfaces entrain room air if the suction applied to the scavenger is too strong. Closed interfaces have negative-pressure relief valves that open and allow room air to enter the system in an effort to not expose the patient to negative pressure in the circuit. There are often two negative-pressure valves on a closed interface system, one set at 0.5 cm H_2O and the other set at 1.8 cm H_2O.

Incorrect Assembly

This would require some effort because the connections for scavengers are of a different size than other connections on an anesthesia machine. That being said, a person without too much knowledge of the proper function and assembly of tubing might think the patient circle circuit attaches to a closed interface because it has a reservoir bag. It is true that it may be far-fetched, but anything can happen. It is hoped the anesthetist would notice such a mistake immediately.

Environmental Concerns

Some worry about the effect that nitrous oxide and the halogenated agents have after they are vented into the atmosphere.

CONCLUSION

We hope you now have a better understanding of the purpose and function of an anesthesia machine scavenger. It is part of the machine that is often overlooked, and even experienced clinicians might not know much about it. It is an integral part of the anesthesia machine and should be part of a daily machine checkout. It should also be monitored frequently during the day to ensure it is doing its job adequately.

FAIL-SAFE SYSTEMS | 11

KEYWORDS

- medical gas cylinders
- alarm and safety features: anesthesia machine
- proportioning devices
- pressure fail-safe

A "fail-safe" is a system or device that limits damage or harm. For instance, on locomotives, there is a "dead man's switch" that the engineer must push every couple of minutes or the train will stop. This is a "fail-safe" in that if the engineer is incapacitated, unconscious, or dead, the train will stop automatically. Another fail-safe is the activation bar on walk-behind lawn mowers. The bar, on the handle of the mower, must be pushed in for the mower blade to spin. If you let go of the bar, the blade stops. *Failsafe* was also a great movie from the 1960s with Henry Fonda. You should watch it. George Clooney remade it in 2000, and it is pretty good, too.

You will find that virtually all fail-safes, whether in anesthesia or in other disciplines or circumstances, are *not* 100% foolproof. They can be intentionally or unintentionally circumvented, or they may malfunction in such a way that the event the fail-safe was supposed to prevent occurs anyway.

Let's use the lawn mower as an example. We said the mower has an activation bar that must be pushed in along the mower handle for the cutting blade to spin. You're mowing the lawn, but you are so tired of how the blade stops every time your hand shifts or you lose your grip. So you decide to tie the activation bar down to the handle, so when you let go to wipe your brow or adjust your iPod, the blade keeps going. You don't have to grip the handle as tightly now because your hands *were* getting tired. You push the mower down a small slope and lose your footing; your foot slips in front of you as you fall backward. Where is your foot going to end up? It's going to end up under the mower, where it will meet a sharp, spinning, hardened steel blade that unfortunately is going to lop off a good part of your foot. If you hadn't tied the blade activation bar down, when you lost your footing and lost your grip on the mower handle, the blade would have stopped quickly enough that you would still have all your toes.

When we discuss fail-safes on an anesthesia machine, it is usually in reference to preventing the delivery of a hypoxic mixture of gas to the patient. These devices usually have something to do with preventing giving the patient too much nitrous oxide versus too little oxygen. They do a good job, but we will discuss later that hypoxic mixtures can still be given to a patient *despite* these built-in fail-safes on anesthesia machines. Fail-safes are found in various places on the anesthesia machine, and we will go over the location and function of each one. Some of them we discuss in other chapters, but will still be discussed here.

CYLINDER COLOR

If your only fail-safe system was this, you would be in trouble. This is a very weak fail-safe and is hardly worth the distinction of being called a fail-safe. It is true, of course, that in the system of coloring in the United States, oxygen is green, nitrous oxide is blue, air is yellow, and so forth. However, remember that this color system varies in different countries. What is more startling is that color coding of medical gas cylinders *is not* a Food and Drug Administration regulation. Color coding is more or less a suggestion and is a weak standard for the medical gas industry. To be legal, cylinders have to be *labeled* correctly but not color coded correctly. Multiple reports of medical gas in different color cylinders have been published, and discovery of an air cylinder that was gray, not yellow, has happened to the authors. In our case, the cylinder was properly labeled and contained the proper gas when analyzed but was the incorrect color.

PIN INDEX SAFETY SYSTEM

The *Pin Index Safety System* is the system that keeps us from putting the incorrect gas cylinder on the incorrect yoke on the back of the anesthesia machine. Each stem of a specific tank has two holes that are in positions that mate with two pins on the appropriate yoke. The holes from an oxygen cylinder do not match up to the pins on the nitrous oxide yoke and vice versa. This is a very good system for ensuring proper placement of gas cylinders on an anesthesia machine. However, misplacement of cylinders is still possible even with the pin index system.

Apart from intentional vandalism, where pins on the yoke were knocked off with a chisel, is it possible to defeat the pin index safety system? The answer is "yes." When replacing a gas cylinder on the back of the machine, only one washer should be placed between the cylinder stem and the yoke nipple. If old washers are not removed, they can act as spacers, and defeat the pin index safety system by not allowing the pins and holes to mate.

DIAMETER INDEX SAFETY SYSTEM

Most people who know about the *Diameter Index Safety System* probably think it refers to the ends of the gas supply hoses that attach to the wall outlets. It is true that these connectors are designed to fit specifically into the correct outlet, but this is *not* the Diameter Index Safety System.

Take a look on the back of your anesthesia machine where the gas hoses enter the machine itself. This is where the diameter index safety system is. Each inlet for each different gas is of a *different diameter*, so the oxygen hose will not fit on the nitrous oxide inlet and vice versa. This system is more fool-proof than the Pin Index Safety System because we rarely if ever disconnect our gas hoses from the machine. Also, to alter the connectors would require deliberate effort.

The main way that this fail-safe system can be defeated is *if the gas supply lines are crossed*. Let's say we have the correct connector from the pipeline source to the gas hose, and we have the correct hose attached to the correct inlet, but if the gas coming out of the pipeline is not oxygen when we think it is, we will be delivering nitrous oxide or air to a patient. Crossed pipelines have happened multiple times in the past, and patients have died because they received a hypoxic gas mixture. After construction work or repair to a medical gas pipeline, each outlet needs to be checked to see if it is delivering the correct gas.

OXYGEN–NITROUS OXIDE FAIL-SAFE VALVE

As you can see, none of the just discussed systems (color-coded cylinders, Pin Index Safety System, and Diameter Index Safety System) are foolproof. Someone could either intentionally or unintentionally defeat them. Also, all three of them are *outside* the anesthesia machine. The *oxygen–nitrous oxide fail-safe valve* is the first fail-safe we will discuss in this chapter that is *inside* the machine. Unlike the previously mentioned systems, you will never see this device unless you open up a machine and go looking for it.

The purpose of this device is to cut off or proportionately decrease nitrous oxide in case oxygen pressure is lost. There are different versions of this device as well. We will discuss the two main types. Keep in mind that one type will have an "all-or-nothing" effect, meaning that if the device senses a decrease in oxygen pressure, nitrous oxide delivery will be blocked. The other

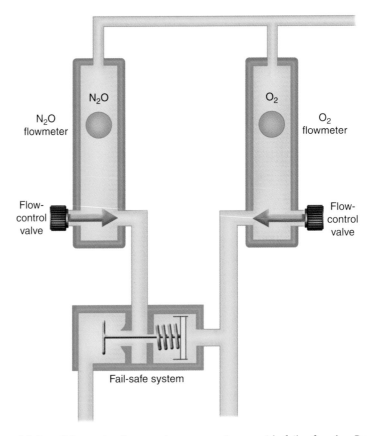

Figure 11-1 ▪ Schematic of a generic oxygen–nitrous oxide fail-safe valve. Depending on the specific type, nitrous oxide delivery will stop completely or proportionately decrease with a decrease in oxygen pressure. (Reproduced with permission from Morgan GE, Mikhail MS, Murray MJ. *Clinical Anesthesiology*. 2nd ed. New York, NY: McGraw-Hill; 2002. Figure 4-3.)

type proportionately decreases nitrous oxide pressure and volume as oxygen pressure and volume are lost (Figure 11-1).

The Datex-Ohmeda type of oxygen–nitrous oxide fail-safe is called a *pressure sensor shutoff valve*. The pressure of the oxygen line inside the machine holds open a spring-loaded valve. This spring-loaded valve sits across the nitrous oxide line. Whenever the pressure of oxygen falls below 20 psig, the spring-loaded valve closes and cuts off the supply of nitrous oxide. This type is an all-or-nothing type device; when the oxygen pressure dips below the threshold of 20 psig, *all* nitrous oxide delivery is stopped. Newer Datex-Ohmeda machines have what is called a *balance regulator*. It works in a similar way, with oxygen pressure holding open a spring-loaded valve, but instead of all-or-nothing nitrous oxide delivery, it proportionately decreases nitrous oxide as oxygen pressure decreases.

The Draeger fail-safe valve is called an *oxygen failure protection device* (OFPD). It works more or less the same as the Datex-Ohmeda balance regulator, allowing for proportionate decreases in nitrous oxide as the oxygen pressure decreases.

These types of fail-safe valves are another example of the simple beauty of machine design: no electronics or sensors are used. They are located between the pressure regulators and the flowmeters in the *intermediate-pressure system*.

OXYGEN–NITROUS OXIDE PROPORTIONING SYSTEMS

In addition to fail-safe valves that protect against a drop of oxygen pressure to the patient, there are means designed to protect the patient from the clinician's dialing in a hypoxic mixture at the point of the flowmeters. These are called *proportioning systems*. As you can probably guess, different companies have different ways of doing this. One type uses a mechanical linkage (traditional Datex-Ohmeda machines). Another type uses a pneumatic pressure system (Draeger). A more sophisticated way is by electronic control (e.g., Datex-Ohmeda ADU).

The kind of system that is found historically in Datex-Ohmeda products is the *Link-25 system*. It is an oxygen ratio controller that links the oxygen and nitrous oxide flowmeters. You have probably seen diagrams of this proportioning system in textbooks. Unlike many things found inside an anesthesia machine, this device looks somewhat familiar to us. It looks like a sprocket chain on a bicycle (Figure 11-2).

The Link-25 system is a *mechanical linkage* between the oxygen and nitrous oxide *flow control valves*. The linkage looks like a sprocket chain, and in fact, the flow control valves have cogs or sprockets on them. The nitrous oxide cog is smaller, with 14 teeth. The oxygen cog has 29 teeth. The two flowmeters can act independently, but when you turn up the nitrous oxide concentration without changing the oxygen flow, the oxygen flow will rise automatically to keep a ratio of about 25% oxygen.

When you turn the nitrous oxide control valve, the sprocket chain turns the oxygen sprocket. But only when you turn the nitrous oxide control valve enough to make the fraction of inspired oxygen (FiO_2) around 25% does a pin on the oxygen sprocket wheel touch a corresponding pin on the oxygen flow control valve and increase the oxygen flow.

The Draeger system at first seems very complex and hard to understand. But if you take a little time to understand it, it too is simple. The Draeger system relies on a pneumatic system, balancing pressures of oxygen and nitrous oxide,

Link-25 proportioning system

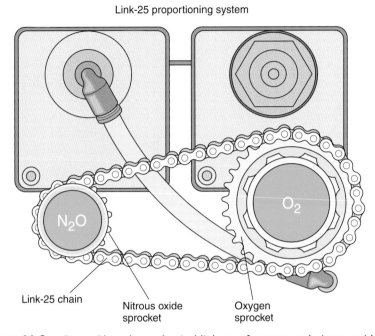

Figure 11-2 ■ Datex-Ohmeda mechanical linkage of oxygen and nitrous oxide gas flows (Link-25). (Reproduced with permission from Morgan GE, Mikhail MS, Murray MJ. *Clinical Anesthesiology.* 4th ed. New York, NY: McGraw-Hill; 2006. Figure 4-16.)

called an *oxygen ratio monitor controller* (ORMC). Newer Draeger machines (e.g., Fabius, Apollo) have a *sensitive oxygen ratio controller* (S-ORC). Both of these devices work similarly and are responsible for closing nitrous oxide delivery in the event of loss of oxygen supply pressure. In our opinion, the ORMC/S-ORC is one of the most difficult devices on an anesthesia machine to understand. We will go slowly in our description and explanation of the basic mechanism of the ORMC (Figure 11-3).

There is a pressurized line that comes off of the *oxygen flow control valve*, which is, in simple terms, the controller at the bottom of the *oxygen flowmeter*. This line ends at a chamber that communicates with a similar chamber that comes off the *nitrous oxide flow control valve*. The gases do not mix. There is a diaphragm for each gas in its specific chamber, and both diaphragms are attached to a rod that moves in response to the relative pressure coming from the diaphragms. At the end of the rod, there is a nitrous oxide *slave valve* (slave because it is tied into the other valves in this system).

The pressure of the oxygen pushes its diaphragm pushes the nitrous oxide diaphragm open, and this also opens the nitrous oxide slave valve, allowing

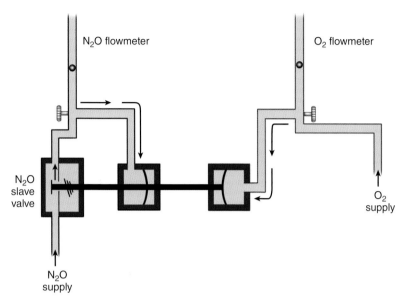

Figure 11-3 ▪ Draeger ORMC. Pressure from the oxygen control valve pushes the oxygen diaphragm to the left, opening the nitrous oxide slave valve, which allows a proportionate flow of nitrous oxide to its flowmeter. The slave valve is spring loaded and allows proportionate flow of nitrous or closes completely of oxygen pressure is lost.

nitrous oxide to flow to it flowmeter, to be available if the clinician chooses to use it. *If* oxygen pressure begins to fall, the nitrous diaphragm will slowly move in proportion to the drop in oxygen pressure. As the nitrous diaphragm moves more, the slave valve for nitrous oxide delivery closes proportionately. When oxygen pressure reaches a certain point, the spring-loaded nitrous oxide slave valve closes completely (Figure 11-4).

The ORMC and its kindred S-ORC control nitrous oxide *in proportion* to oxygen pressure. The system slowly and proportionately lowers nitrous delivery to the flow control valve of the nitrous oxide flowmeter in response to decreased oxygen pressure. As long as there is oxygen pressure, the ORMC will allow some nitrous oxide to reach its flowmeter.

At the flowmeters, increasing the oxygen flow rate increases the pressure inside the oxygen chamber of the ORMC or S-ORC. This allows the slave valve to open more and allows more nitrous oxide to be available at the flowmeter (it doesn't mean that the nitrous oxide will be added to your FGF, simply that it is available for you to use). If you decide to use nitrous oxide, when you open its flowmeter, the pressure in the nitrous oxide chamber of the ORMC causes the nitrous oxide diaphragm to push against the oxygen diaphragm. As the

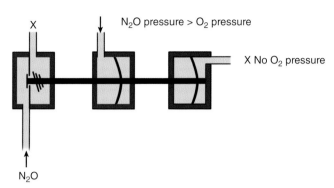

Figure 11-4 ▪ With no oxygen pressure, nitrous diaphragm pushes the rod to the right, closing the nitrous oxide slave valve to block delivery of nitrous oxide to its flowmeter.

nitrous oxide pressure increases and approaches the oxygen pressure, the rod to the slave valve moves, decreasing the nitrous oxide flow.

This system allows continuous feedback, comparing the pressure of nitrous oxide versus oxygen, and keeping delivery of nitrous oxide to the flowmeter at a level that will *not cause* a hypoxic mixture. The illustrations in Figures 11-3 and 11-4 will help you understand better.

The ORMC and S-ORC therefore perform two tasks: they shut off nitrous oxide in the event of oxygen pressure loss and they keep the proportion of oxygen and nitrous oxide so that FiO_2 stays above 0.25 when the flowmeters are used.

Electronic control of gas proportioning will likely be seen more and more commonly as anesthesia machine evolution progresses. Newer Datex-Ohmeda machines have this kind of proportioning system, as do Maquet anesthesia machines. Electronic control is more precise. Also, unlike mechanical and pneumatic linkages, whose actions are at the flowmeters, electronic proportioning also senses and controls FiO_2 downstream of the vaporizers after the addition of inhalational agent. The big advantage to electronic proportioning is that it takes into account the change in FiO_2 caused by addition of inhalational agents. For instance, if you have an FiO_2 of 0.25 and switch from sevoflurane to desflurane as your inhalational agent, your oxygen concentration will likely drop to below 0.21 if you need 1 minimum alveolar concentration (MAC) of desflurane. An electronic proportioning system senses the FiO_2 after the agent has been added to the fresh gas flow (FGF) and would therefore increase the amount of oxygen in the FGF to keep from delivering a hypoxic mixture. But unlike the previously mentioned mechanical and pneumatic systems, the electronic control will not work without some source of power, either from the wall outlets or from its own backup battery source.

HAZARDS OF FAIL-SAFE VALVES, ORMC, S-ORC, AND LINK-25

As we continue to say, these devices are not *foolproof*. A hypoxic mixture could still reach the patient in the following ways if no other fail-safes or monitors closer to the patient existed:

1. Gas supply lines could be crossed, so oxygen is actually not coming out of the oxygen line.
2. Tank supplies could be mismatched, with wrong tanks on the wrong yoke through a failure of the Pin Index Safety System.
3. Gas supply hoses could be going into the wrong machine connector through a failure of the Diameter Index Safety System.
4. Another gas could be added into the FGF (e.g., helium). There are no fail-safes connecting nitrous oxide and helium delivery if a machine has ability to deliver helium.
5. Leaks in the flowmeter system, leaving an FGF with low levels of oxygen
6. Addition of desflurane to an FGF that is very close to an FiO_2 of 0.21
7. Malfunction of the oxygen ratio controller
8. Circuit disconnect

This is why anesthesia machines have other means of detecting hypoxic mixtures, downstream of these devices, namely, an oxygen sensor at the beginning of the inspiratory limb of the circuit and inspired and end-tidal oxygen gas monitoring.

Some machines, but not all, do not allow you to turn the oxygen flow off totally. The lowest flow in these machines is 250 mL/min.

CONCLUSION

We hope you now know more about anesthesia machine fail-safe devices than you did previously. We also hope you see that *none of them are foolproof.* There is no substitute for an alert, vigilant anesthesiologist or anesthetist.

ELECTRICAL SYSTEMS | 12

KEYWORDS

- design and ergonomics of anesthesia machines
- electrical safety features
- anesthesia machine

Although early anesthesia machines did not require any electrical power, those made in the last several decades do rely on electricity for various functions. As machines have changed and become more complex, more and more systems on anesthesia machines depend on an external power source. Fortunately for us and our patients, the most vital functions of most anesthesia machines still do not require electricity. Do you know what parts of the anesthesia machine or machines that you commonly use would still work if electrical power were lost?

In this chapter, we will discuss things in *generalities* because not all anesthesia machines will operate the same way in case of a power outage. When electrical power is lost, what may work on one model of machine may not work on another model even from the same manufacturer. We will discuss the basic components of the electrical system of an anesthesia machine and what to do in the event of a power loss during an anesthetic.

The basic components of the electrical system of an anesthesia machine include a master switch, electrical outlets, circuit breakers, and (in most cases) a backup power source. The most modern machines also have data ports that allow information to pass between the machine display and various monitors.

MASTER SWITCH

This switch does two things: it turns on the *electrical system*, and it activates the *pneumatic system*. Although we call it a switch, it can be a knob, a switch, or even a button, depending on the model. When turned on, all of the electrical components of the machine are powered up. (This may or may not include patient monitors, again, depending on the model and setup.) In addition, the pneumatic system of the machine is activated. There is an electronic valve in the pneumatic system that, when opened by the master switch, allows communication between the gas sources (pipeline or cylinders) and the rest of the machine. The reason for this is that when you turn off the machine, gas is not left on and wasted.

The important thing to remember about the master switch is that even if there is no electricity, as long as the master switch is *turned on*, the pneumatic system will work. On some more modern machines, however, if you have been on backup battery power for long enough to drain the batteries, the machine's pneumatic system will cease to function when the batteries in fact go dead. In any circumstance, if the master switch is not turned on, the pneumatic system will not work, with one exception: the oxygen flush button bypasses the master switch pneumatic control, so even if the machine master switch is not turned on, the oxygen flush *will* work (Figure 12-1).

❘ ELECTRICAL OUTLETS

On most machines, there is a set of electrical outlets on the back of the machine. These are there for one reason: to provide a convenient way to plug in the patient monitors if the monitors are not an integral part of the anesthesia machine. That way, all you have to do is to plug in the single anesthesia machine cord to the wall outlet and not have to plug in all of your monitors.

It seems, however, that the presence of these outlets is a powerful attractant to other operating room (OR) personnel. Even the baby-proof plug-in shields are not a deterrent. Imagine there is someone trying to find a place to plug in a cautery machine, or a warmer, or the OR table, or the patient bed. "Hey, there's some plug-ins right back here on the anesthesia machine!" they think. With no malice intended, they plug in whatever they want to plug in, and at some time during the case, suddenly and with no warning, your anesthesia machine goes dead—the ventilator just stops. Your monitors go dead, too, if they are part of the machine or plugged into the back of the machine.

At some time in your career, this will happen to you. It has happened to the authors multiple times. You need to know immediately how to troubleshoot and figure out the problem. You may say, "But doesn't the machine have a battery backup?" Maybe it does, and maybe it doesn't. You'd better find out. One of the authors had anesthesia machine power loss *with* a machine that had an internal battery backup. The battery, it turned out, was old enough that it didn't hold a charge. It was a model of machine that did not show a screen icon indicating proper battery function.

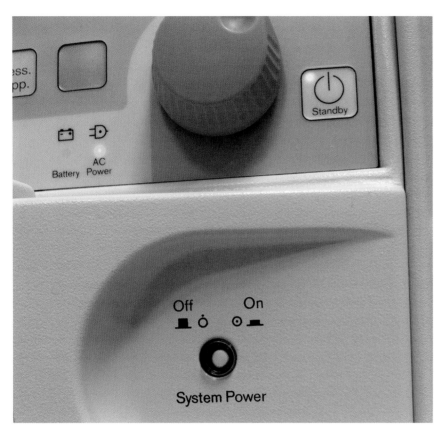

Figure 12-1 ▪ Master switch on a Draeger Apollo anesthesia machine. When engaged, both the electrical *and* pneumatic systems become operational. Note the AC power and battery icons in the upper left of the figure; AC (wall outlet) is supplying power in this case (the AC icon is lit).

In the case of a machine that *does* have an auxiliary power source, the machine will let you know by visual and auditory cues that you are not on backup power.

In this situation, not only do you need to know *how* to fix the problem, you also need to know *what functions of the machine are going to work* while you are fixing the problem; more on that later. Never let anyone plug anything into your machine unless you are sure they know what they're doing.

So what do you do when this happens? The first thing to do is call for help. You can do this simultaneously as you begin to ventilate and monitor the patient. We will talk about ventilation and monitoring options in this scenario later in the chapter. You need to ask if anyone has plugged *anything* into the back of your machine. You need to ask what the last thing in the room that was plugged in or the last piece of electrical equipment that was used. You need to unplug whatever was recently plugged into the back of your machine or whatever the last piece of electrical equipment in the room that was plugged in or used. You need to reset the circuit breakers.

Notice that we said to find out not only if anything was plugged into the back of your machine, but also the last thing plugged into any outlet in the room and the last electrical device used in the room. There are a lot of things that draw a lot of current, and your machine circuit breakers can trip from something else in the room that is in use. Furthermore, we have seen a case when the machine died while the nurse still had her hand on the plug behind the machine, and we have seen a case when the fluoroscope that a surgery resident plugged into the back of the machine without our knowledge had been in use for about an hour before the machine died. A situation like this is one when extra hands and brains are necessary. Someone has to care for the patient while the mess is being straightened out.

CIRCUIT BREAKERS

Do you know where the circuit breakers are on the machine or machines that you commonly use? If not, you'd better find out because just like we mentioned in the last section, at some time in your career, a circuit breaker on your machine *will* trip. Even if the machine's battery backup works, you need to know what to do and where the circuit breakers are (because the battery backup could possibly not activate). Unfortunately, there is no industry standard for where the circuit breakers will be found. Usually, they are on the back of the machine, but they can be hard to see, small and unobtrusive, or hidden behind a roll of cables. At least one model of machine had its circuit breakers on the front of the machine over the vaporizers. For a specialty that is so interested in safety, nonstandard placement of circuit breakers is one glaring oversight in our opinion.

BATTERY BACKUP

Most modern anesthesia machines have a battery backup in the event electrical power from the wall is lost. Most also have some type of icon or message that tells the operator the percent charge on the battery and if the battery is actually in use. For machines that do not have a battery backup, reserve or auxiliary power units (APUs) are available for use. These are readily available and can be easily attached to an anesthesia machine, and they will last a longer period of time than the built-in backup power source would last if electrical power is lost.

How long will your backup battery last? That question depends on several variables such as the type of battery, use of mechanical ventilation, how many systems in the anesthesia machine are dependent on electricity, if patient monitors are using the same battery, and so forth. Depending on these variables, the machine, and the battery, the time period can be anywhere from half an hour to 2 hours. It is your responsibility to find out approximately how long the machine or machines you use can last on their batteries.

SO WHAT WORKS WHEN ALL THE POWER IS GONE?

Again, that question depends on the machine. Most machines (we know we have said "most machines" quite a bit in this chapter, but there are a lot of different models of anesthesia machines out there, and they are not all the same), even with their modern complexities, are still designed to be able to deliver oxygen to a patient as long as the master switch is turned on and there is a source of oxygen attached to the machine. The circle circuit still works, the reservoir bag still works, the adjustable pressure-limiting (APL) valve still works, the unidirectional valves still work, and the carbon dioxide absorber still works. Therefore, you can ventilate a patient manually, or the patient can breathe spontaneously. Again, we said "most machines." You really need to find out for yourself what your specific machine would do without electricity.

Do the flowmeters still work? If your machine has standard glass, Thorpe tube flowmeters with nonelectronic controls and knobs you turn instead of electronic selection, they probably do. What about machines with "virtual flowmeters" (flowmeters on an LCD screen)? Maybe. For instance, the Draeger Apollo, which has virtual flowmeters, still has a small glass Thorpe tube flowmeter on the front of the machine under the LCD screen for use if the screen goes dead. It measures all three gases, not just oxygen, but it does give you an indication of the flow rate through the machine, so it would be better to use only oxygen in such a situation. The flowmeter control knobs on the Apollo are mechanical.

How would you keep the patient anesthetized? You could switch from inhalational to an intravenous technique if you had been using the vaporizers. But would the vaporizers still work? Probably, yes. If the vaporizer was a standard variable bypass flow-over type that required no electricity in the first place, the answer is yes. If it is a desflurane "vaporizer," the answer is no because we know that the desflurane vaporizer needs electricity to heat and pressurize the agent, plus relies on electronics to inject the liquid into the fresh gas flow. Also, Maquet injection-type units would not work. Plus, the vaporizer system on the Ohmeda ADU with its external cassettes and internal vaporizing mechanism will not function without electricity. The ADU needs power for its flowmeters also. At our institution, we have some ADU machines and auxiliary power units are installed on each one.

FUNCTIONS OF A STANDARD ANESTHESIA MACHINE NOT NEEDING ELECTRICITY TO FUNCTION

This is provided the master switch is in the "on" position.

1. Oxygen delivery
2. Nitrous oxide delivery
3. Medical air delivery
4. Oxygen–nitrous oxide failsafe valve
5. Oxygen–nitrous oxide proportioning systems
6. Oxygen flush button
7. Mechanical flowmeter control knobs
8. Glass flowmeters
9. Variable bypass flow over vaporizers (e.g., Tec, Draeger 2000, Penlon Sigma Delta)
10. APL valve
11. Unidirectional circle circuit valves
12. Reservoir bag
13. Circle circuit
14. Carbon dioxide absorber
15. Scavenger system (provided the wall vacuum is unaffected)

If your machine does not appear to be working properly, grab your bag valve mask (BVM). That is why, of course, you should have a BVM on the back of your cart or machine at all times. It is your backup anesthesia machine. You would need to switch to an intravenous technique as well. Also tell the surgeons to hurry up. This isn't the time to let the intern close.

How would you monitor the patient? A spare transport monitor would be great in this circumstance. Let's hope there is one nearby and that the power outage isn't throughout the whole OR because then spare transport monitors would be pretty scarce.

What are some other ways to monitor the patient? There are certain practices that we as a specialty have gotten away from because of the sophistication of patient monitoring. These include a finger on the pulse, auscultation, looking at nail beds for color, and so forth. Don't think we are advocating not using monitors—of course not! But it is true that the more we rely on our monitors, the less we touch the patient.

WHAT THE FUTURE HOLDS

Improved features in anesthesia machine design and anesthetic delivery, for the most part, require electricity of some sort to work, whether external (power outlet), or internal (battery backup). Already, some commonly used vaporizers need electricity to function. Electronic oxygen–nitrous oxide proportioning systems will become increasingly more common. "Virtual" or electronic flowmeters are common now as well. We will leave it up to you to decide if "newer" means "better" in all cases. But like it or not, features found on anesthesia machines that do not need electricity to function will become less common over the next few years.

CONCLUSION

This chapter has shown that there can be quite a bit of difference in how anesthesia machines function or do not function when there is a lack of electricity. You have also seen by our example that even if a machine has a backup battery, the battery can malfunction or be dead at the moment it is needed. In addition, you have seen that it is necessary to have a plan of action when a power outage occurs during an anesthetic case. It is ultimately your responsibility to know what would happen to the machine or machines that you commonly use when electrical supply is disrupted. In times of crisis in the OR, most personnel turn to the anesthesia provider. It is up to you to be prepared.

ANESTHESIA MACHINE CHECKOUT | 13

KEYWORDS

- design and ergonomics of anesthesia machines
- anesthesia machine safety features
- ventilators
- oxygen
- ASA monitoring standards

In the recent past, it was easier to perform a preanesthetic checkout on an anesthesia machine. The machines were not as complicated, and the checkout did not differ much from one type of machine to another. There was a list that you could either commit to memory or attach to the machine as a guide, and you had to complete each step, similar to an airline pilot's preflight checkout. (But as we said earlier, we anesthesia providers would be much more careful about machine checkout if not only the patient's, but *our* lives depended on it, in the same way a pilot's life depends on his or her machine.)

Things are much different now. Not only are there many more models of anesthesia machines, with different features, but some machines do an *automated* checkout. This makes things potentially confusing because an automated checkout may or may not check for everything that needs to be checked. As an example, the user manual for some machines will indicate that the user is to perform a low-pressure leak test, but other machines do not. It can certainly be difficult to remember what machine requires what test to be performed by the user instead of being done automatically by the machine. The manufacturers say the clinician needs to read the user manual, and certainly that is true, but few of us do or even know where to find one. In fact, there is now not a standard preanesthesia checkout for every machine because machines vary so much. In 2008, the American Society of Anesthesiologists

(ASA) devised an overview[1] of what should be checked, but not in the "step one, step two" manner of previous checklists.

Keep in mind that a failure to perform a complete preanesthetic machine checkout would not be looked upon favorably in a medicolegal situation if any untoward event led to patient injury related to an equipment malfunction. But besides that, it is of prime importance that we as caregivers strive to perform at the highest standards possible; clinical excellence is not to be hoped for but is to be expected.

STANDARD MACHINE CHECKOUT

So, what is part of a standard anesthesia machine checkout? Sadly, the only morning checkout many clinicians will perform is to simply see if the anesthesia circle circuit will hold positive pressure. In an emergency situation, that may indeed be all that you have time to do. If a patient may suffer because of a delay, a machine check of the most basic things is appropriate; this would include if the power is on, if a source of oxygen is attached, and if the circuit hold can positive pressure.

Table 13-1 provides a generic machine checkout list from the Food and Drug Administration that has been used for many years. It is still quite adaptable to many anesthesia machines. Even with machines that have an automated checkout system, this list can be referenced for things that may not be checked by the automatic system. For instance, an automated system will not tell you if you have suction, airway equipment, or a bag valve mask (BVM; "Ambu") available.

Keep in mind that this checkout list is for a bellows ventilator, but nevertheless it can be modified for use with a piston-type ventilator anesthesia machine or for a bellows machine with an automated checkout. Some newer machines may not have an outlet from where to perform a low-pressure test. That is where you need to know what is in the user manual from the manufacturer and what it recommends in such a situation.

AUTOMATED MACHINE CHECKOUT

Whether it is called automated, automatic, or electronic, this kind of checkout is a mixed blessing in our opinion. Although it can check out the sophisticated electronics of modern anesthesia machines better than we can and will never miss a step, it *may or may not* be an inclusive checkout, depending on the type of machine. Even though we call it automated, many of the machines with an automated checkout still require a human operator during the process to

Table 13-1 **ANESTHESIA APPARATUS CHECKOUT RECOMMENDATIONS**

Emergency ventilation equipment

1. Verify backup ventilation equipment is available and functioning.*

High-pressure system

2. Check O_2 cylinder supply.*
   a. Open O_2 cylinder and verify at least half full (about 1000 psig).
   b. Close cylinder
3. Check central pipeline supplies; check that hoses are connected and pipeline gauges read about 50 psig.*

Low-pressure system

4. Check initial status of low-pressure system.*
   a. Close flow control valves and turn off vaporizers.
   b. Check fill level and tighten vaporizers' filler caps.
5. Perform leak check of machine low-pressure system.*
   a. Verify that the machine master switch and flow control valves are off.
   b. Attach suction bulb to common (fresh) gas outlet.
   c. Squeeze bulb repeatedly until fully collapsed.
   d. Verify bulb stays *fully* collapsed for at least 10 seconds.
   e. Open one vaporizer at a time and repeat steps c and d.
   f. Remove suction bulb and reconnect fresh gas hose.
6. Turn on machine master switch and all other necessary electrical equipment.*
7. Test flowmeters.*
   a. Adjust flow of all gases through their full range, checking for smooth operation of floats and undamaged flow tubes.
   b. Attempt to create a hypoxic O_2/N_2O mixture and verify correct changes in flow and/or alarm.

Scavenging system

8. Adjust and check scavenging system.*
   a. Ensure proper connections between the scavenging system and both APL (pop-off) valve and ventilator relief valve.
   b. Adjust waste-gas vacuum (if possible).
   c. Fully open APL valve and occlude Y piece.
   d. With minimum O_2 flow, allow scavenger reservoir bag to collapse completely and verify that absorber pressure gauge reads about zero.
   e. With the O_2 flush activated, allow scavenger reservoir bag to distend fully, and then verify that absorber pressure gauge reads <10 cm H_2O.

Breathing system

9. Calibrate O_2 monitor.*
   a. Ensure monitor reads 21% in room air.
   b. Verify low-O_2 alarm is enabled and functioning.
   c. Reinstall sensor in circuit and flush breathing system with O_2.
   d. Verify that monitor now reads greater than 90%.

(continued)

Table 13-1   ANESTHESIA APPARATUS CHECKOUT RECOMMENDATIONS (*continued*)

10. Check initial status breathing system.
    a. Set selector switch to bag mode.
    b. Check that breathing circuit is complete, undamaged, and unobstructed.
    c. Verify that CO_2 absorbent is adequate.
    d. Install breathing-circuit accessory equipment (e.g., humidifier, PEEP valve) to be used during the case.
11. Perform leak check of the breathing system.
    a. Set all gas flows to zero (or minimum).
    b. Close APL (pop-off) valve and occlude Y piece.
    c. Pressurize breathing system to about 30 cm H_2O with O_2 flush.
    d. Ensure that pressure remains fixed for at least 10 seconds.
    e. Open APL (pop-off) valve and ensure that pressure decreases.

Manual and automatic ventilation systems

12. Test ventilation systems and unidirectional valves.
    a. Place a second breathing bag on Y piece.
    b. Set appropriate ventilator parameters for next patient.
    c. Switch to automatic-ventilation (ventilator) mode.
    d. Turn ventilator on and fill bellows and breathing bag with O_2 flush.
    e. Set O_2 flow to minimum, other gas flows to zero.
    f. Verify that during inspiration bellows deliver appropriate tidal volume and that during expiration bellows fill completely.
    g. Set fresh gas flow to about 5 L min^{-1}.
    h. Verify that the ventilator bellows and simulated lungs fill and empty appropriately without sustained pressure at end expiration.
    i. *Check for proper action of unidirectional valves.*
    j. Exercise breathing circuit accessories to ensure proper function.
    k. Turn ventilator off and switch to manual ventilation (bag/APL) mode.
    l. Ventilate manually and ensure inflation and deflation of artificial lungs and appropriate feel of system resistance and compliance.
    m. Remove second breathing bag from Y piece.

Monitors

13. Check, calibrate, and/or set alarm limits of all monitors: capnograph, pulse oximeter, O_2 analyzer, respiratory-volume monitor (spirometer), pressure monitor with high and low airway-pressure alarms.

(*continued*)

Table 13-1   **ANESTHESIA APPARATUS CHECKOUT RECOMMENDATIONS** (*continued*)

Final position

14. Check final status of machine.
   a. Vaporizers off
   b. APL valve open
   c. Selector switch to bag mode
   d. All flowmeters to zero (or minimum)
   e. Patient suction level adequate
   f. Breathing system ready to use

APL, adjustable pressure-limiting; PEEP, positive end-expiratory pressure.

*If an anesthesia provider uses the same machine in successive cases, these steps need not be repeated, or they can be abbreviated after the initial checkout.

Reproduced with permission from Morgan GE, Mikhail MS, Murray MJ. *Clinical Anesthesiology*. 4th ed. New York, NY: McGraw-Hill; 2006.

open or close valves and so forth by following instructions on the interface screen. And still, it moves the operator one more step away from the process of machine checkout, and with that, removes the operator from thinking about and understanding how the machine works. It moves the anesthesia machine closer to the concept of a "black box," something that the user is not supposed to know how it works. An anesthesia machine with automated checkout keeps track of how often the complete checkout was performed.

Because it is not possible to have a universal checkout for modern machines because of design and feature differences and the amount of automation in self-testing, the ASA's "Recommendations for Pre-Anesthesia Checkout Procedures" is a useful guideline even though it is much less specific than the previous standard anesthesia machine checkout list.[1] Steps in the list below marked with an asterisk (*) are done only in the morning *or* if the machine is moved from one location to another; the other steps are done between each case.

1. **Verify that the auxiliary oxygen cylinder and self-inflating manual ventilation device are available and functioning.***

   An electronic preanesthesia checkout cannot discern if there is a BVM (Ambu), which is your *backup anesthesia machine*, is there or not.

2. **Verify whether patient suction is adequate to clear a patient airway.***

   Suction might very well be the thing that is forgotten the most during a room setup; the buckets and controls are probably behind the machine and hard to get to, the tubing may not be long enough, and so forth. Also, is the suction *strong enough*? Some things we still have to do ourselves instead of having the automated checkout do it.

3. **Turn on the anesthesia delivery system and confirm that AC power is available.**[*]

It is possible, as one of the authors embarrassingly discovered while he was a resident, to do an anesthesia circuit pressure check with the oxygen flush button with the electric power to the machine turned off. The flush button works when electric power is off, but the rest of the pneumatic system does not.

4. **Verify availability of required monitors and check the alarms.**

Have you ever been setting up your room and not noticed there were no electrocardiographic leads until the patient was in the room? Again, an automated machine checkout will not tell you something like that. As far as alarms, did the last clinician turn off the alarms? Are they set where you want them? Are you doing an adult, pediatric, or neonatal case?

5. **Verify that pressure is adequate on the spare oxygen cylinder mounted on the anesthesia machine.**[*]

This may or may not be part of an automated anesthesia machine checkout; some machines may prompt the user to open the cylinder to check pressure, but others may not.

6. **Verify that piped gas pressures are equal to or greater than 50 psig.**[*]

We always assume there is enough pipeline pressure, but assumption can be a bad thing.

7. **Verify that vaporizers are adequately filled, and if applicable, that filler ports are tightly closed.**[*]

Desflurane vaporizers will indicate if filling is necessary, but in general, common vaporizers do not. That is up to you; it is the same with closing up vaporizers after filling.

8. **Verify that there are no leaks in the gas supply lines between the flowmeters and the common gas outlet.**[*]

This may be done by your machine or not. If not, how to perform this varies from machine to machine, so instruction from a manufacturer's representative, biomedical technician, colleague, or user manual is necessary. An old-fashioned negative leak test may be needed (see step 4 in Table 13-1). In addition, leaks from unclosed vaporizers will not be detected unless that vaporizer was turned on.

9. **Test scavenging system function.**[*]

Whether the machine has an open or closed interface, the scavenger system needs to be checked. Is the scavenger attached to vacuum? Is the vacuum hose unobstructed? Unfortunately, some machine designs make it difficult to adjust scavenger suction. The flowmeter for an open interface system may be in the back of the machine, not visible from the usual user's position.

10. **Calibrate, or verify the calibration, of the oxygen monitor and check the low oxygen alarm.**

    Some oxygen sensors require the user to calibrate the sensor to room air; other designs are self-calibrating.

11. **Verify that carbon dioxide absorbent is not exhausted.**

    Absorbent status, whether it is good, exhausted, or even present, is not checked automatically. If you some in on Monday morning and the anesthesia machine was left on all weekend, think about changing the absorbent even if it does not look exhausted; it may be desiccated (more on that in the carbon dioxide absorber Chapter 9). Also, do you trust the person who refilled the canister? The absorber is a common place for leaks.

12. **Perform breathing system pressure and leak testing.**

    This is part of many automated checkouts. The circuit is also checked for its compliance automatically on some machines, so the circuit should be the way you intend to use it, whether partially or completely extended. The machine will have greater accuracy in set versus delivered tidal volume because the circuit's compliance will be factored into volume delivery.

13. **Verify that gas flows properly through breathing circuit during both inspiration and exhalation.**

    This can be done by breathing through the circuit or using a spare reservoir bag or a specialty reservoir. Leak testing will not necessarily detect an *obstruction* to ventilation. This can be a concern with coaxial circle circuits because the inspired limb is not clearly seen.

14. **Document completion of checkout procedures.**

    Documentation may be done automatically by the machine. Most machines keep a log of checks, and this information can be retrieved if needed. Many anesthetic written or automated records also have a check box indicating that the anesthesia machine was checked out properly.

15. **Confirm the ventilator settings and evaluate readiness to deliver anesthesia care.**

    You do not want to turn on the ventilator for a pediatric patient, having not changed the tidal volume setting for the adult you just anesthetized. Some call this step an "anesthetic time-out," making sure that you are ready to deliver a safe anesthetic, with not only a proper anesthesia machine and monitoring setup but also to ensure you are prepared for airway management, medication delivery, line setups, and so forth.

CONCLUSION

Who checks the machine? In some practices, properly trained and certified anesthesia technicians are involved with machine setup and checkout, not only in the morning but also between cases. Biomedical technicians also may be trained to perform preanesthetic checkouts. Ultimately, however, it is the responsibility of the anesthesia provider or provider team to make sure the machine and room itself are ready to provide an anesthetic. That is why *you* need to know how to do a machine check out and why you need to know how an anesthesia machine works.

REFERENCE

1. American Society of Anesthesiologists. 2008 ASA Recommendations for Pre-Anesthesia Checkout. http://www.asahq.org/For-Members/Clinical-Information/2008-ASA-Recommendations-for-PreAnesthesia-Checkout.aspx. Published 2008. Accessed February 8, 2013.

MALIGNANT HYPERTHERMIA AND THE ANESTHESIA MACHINE

14

KEYWORDS

- malignant hyperthermia
- nontriggering anesthetics
- filters
- design and ergonomics of anesthesia machines

Malignant hyperthermia (MH) is "the disease of anesthesia." We are the only specialty that until recently needed to know anything about it. That is changing with time as more episodes of "awake triggering" not related to anesthesia are being reported. Nevertheless, MH is a condition that the overwhelming majority of us will never see, but we need to be able to recognize and treat it immediately.

In this chapter, we wish not to discuss the diagnosis and treatment of MH as such. You will find that covered thoroughly in the major anesthesia textbooks. What we want to discuss is how to prepare an anesthesia machine preoperatively for a patient who is at risk for MH and what to do with an anesthesia machine during an anesthetic in which a patient develops MH. So, what do we need to do to our machine in such a circumstance?

Anesthesia machines were much simpler in the past. And because they were simpler, it was much easier to make them safe to use on an MH-susceptible patient. All you needed to do was to flush the machine with high fresh gas flow (FGF), usually by running the bellows ventilator at a high tidal volume and FGF, with a reservoir bag on the circuit acting as "lungs." After doing this for 20 to 30 minutes, you changed the circuit and the carbon dioxide absorbent granules, took off the vaporizers (or emptied them and taped the dials closed), and proceeded. Maybe you also unscrewed the clear bellows dome and put a new bellows piece on as well. Studies showed that halogenated anesthetic agent concentrations were very low, less than 5 ppm, which was considered acceptable.

But, of course, anesthesia machines are more complicated now. More parts and pieces of tubing are made of plastic, which can absorb and slowly release anesthetic agent. More complicated gas flow pathways can mean that there are nooks and crannies that are not blown out well during the high FGF flushing process even after a 30-minute flush. So then, after induction of anesthesia, when the FGF is decreased to a level you would use for a case, these unflushed areas will potentially add more molecules of inhalational agent to the FGF in what you thought was a clean machine, therefore increasing the patient's exposure to triggers. This has been called a "rebound effect," when after a long flushing, the concentration of inhalational agent increases because of the release of agent from plastic components and from those areas of the internal circuit that were poorly flushed.

In previous times, the best, safest, and most efficient way to have a machine ready for a nontriggering anesthetic was to have one anesthesia machine that was "dedicated" as your MH machine. So a brand new machine or one that had been thoroughly flushed and prepared was only used for MH-susceptible patients. This machine would not even have vaporizers installed on it. As long as nobody mistakenly used this machine to deliver inhalational agents, everything was fine.

Now, however, the easiest way to prepare a machine for an MH patient is the use of Vapor-Clean filters (Dynasthetics, Salt Lake City, UT) (Figure 14-1). These single-patient-use activated charcoal filters, one on each limb of the circle circuit, reduce agent concentrations to 5 ppm or less after a 90-second flush, according to the manufacturer. They can be used after a diagnosis of MH is made during a case as well, rapidly decreasing the agent concentration after the agent is discontinued. In a situation of a patient who is exhaling agent, the manufacturer recommends changing the filters after one hour of use. Otherwise, in a situation when no agent had been used, the filters are recommended to be changed after 12 hours of use. The cost of a two-filter kit is in the $70 to $100 range. For a small department or hospital, this is much more cost-efficient than having a dedicated MH machine. The Malignant Hyperthermia Association of the United States (MHAUS) has said that Vapor-Clean filters may be used as an alternative or as an addition to their recommended machine preparation guidelines.

A dedicated MH machine is still a good answer for a large group, department, or hospital where such a machine would be needed more frequently than a smaller institution, especially because capital funds have already been used to obtain and maintain the machine. However, we think that if subsequent

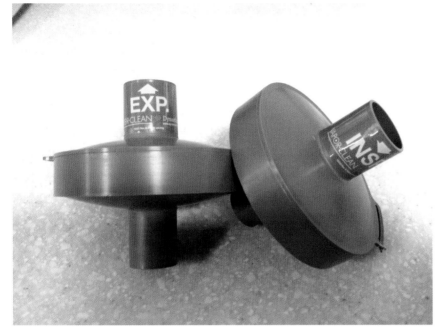

Figure 14-1 ▪ Set of Vapor-Clean filters (Dynasthetics, Salt Lake City UT). Each kit has two filters, one for the inspiratory and one for the expiratory limbs of anesthesia circuit.

studies confirm the initial data concerning Vapor-Clean, there will be no need for dedicated MH machines in the future as long as an institution has an adequate supply of these special filters.

The GE Ohmeda Aisys View has a novel feature that allows the operator to prepare for a nontriggering anesthetic. The whole "left side" or ventilatory section of the machine (everything distal to the common gas outlet) detaches in a matter of seconds to allow replacement with an inhalational agent exposure-free identical section. These replaceable sections are very lightweight and easy to handle. This solves the problem of agent exposure because everything, including the carbon dioxide absorber, has been changed to a component that is agent exposure free. Obviously, you need to have the extra ventilatory section on hand and never expose it to inhalational agents. There is a small section of tubing from the vaporizers to the common gas outlet that is not replaced by a new section, but because it is short and devoid of nooks and crannies, it should be able to be flushed clean of agent quickly.

The bottom line is we cannot recommend for you what to do to prepare your machine for an MH-susceptible patient because it all depends on the circumstances of the situation and what kind of machine you have. Other possibilities include Mapleson circuits, most familiarly the Bain circuit, bag valve mask, a critical care ventilator (all with a total intravenous general anesthetic), or regional anesthesia. But even with regional or monitored anesthesia care, you must, of course, be ready to instantly ventilate a patient. There is no substitute for proper planning.

SUGGESTED READINGS

1. Malignant Hyperthermia Association of the United States. http://www.mhaus.org/healthcare-professionals/mhaus-recommendations/anesthesia-workstation-preparation. Accessed April 18, 2013.
2. Berganheier N, Stoker R, Westensow D, Orr J. Activated charcoal effectively removes inhaled anesthetics from modern anesthesia machines. Anesth Analg 2011;112:1363–1370.

ANESTHESIA EQUIPMENT FOR MAGNETIC RESONANCE IMAGING

15

KEYWORDS

- anesthesia in remote locations
- anesthesia monitoring
- magnetic resonance imaging anesthetic implications and management

There are several anesthetic concerns for magnetic resonance imaging (MRI). Anesthesia providers in general do not like to go anywhere outside of our domain, the operating room (OR), to provide anesthetics. In fact, for years now at our institution, we have called it "going on safari." However, anesthetic provision in remote locations is becoming more and more common as increasing numbers of therapeutic and diagnostic procedures are performed outside of the OR. Complicated procedures require akinesis, often for long periods, as well as life support and even resuscitation, and the best and safest way to meet those needs is with anesthetic care.

Besides being out of our comfort zone, such remote locations can be difficult places to provide anesthesia, owing to room size, darkness, a lack of knowledge by hospital staff as to our needs, provision of medical gases, suction, and the like. On top of that the environment can be potentially hazardous, owing to different types of radiation, so hazardous that we must sometimes monitor the patient from another area by video monitoring.

In the case of MRI, we must deal with issues of anesthesia equipment concerns. Not all anesthesia equipment is "MRI safe"; that is, equipment made from ferromagnetic material can not only interfere with the quality of the MRI image but also damage the patient, personnel, or equipment if it is in the magnetic field of the MRI, causing the equipment to become a projectile. Incidents during which gas cylinders, for instance, along with other pieces of metallic items that may have made their way into the MRI room itself have commonly been reported as causing patient injury, even death, from the great pull of the MRI magnet. In addition to injury from objects flying into the magnetic field causing injury, burns to the patient can also occur from the use of standard monitoring cables, pads, and probes.

So how can we actually monitor a patient in the MRI suite? Fortunately, there is anesthesia equipment and monitoring that is available that will minimize any chance of patient injury, and also not interfere with the MRI image. The purpose of this chapter is not to discuss techniques of providing anesthesia for MRI, but to show how this specialized equipment is "MRI compatible."

| VENTILATION

The simplest way to provide ventilation to a patient undergoing an MRI is with spontaneous ventilation. A bag valve mask (BVM) can be used to provide positive-pressure ventilation by an endotracheal tube or supraglottic device; masking a patient in an MRI would prove difficult because of access problems. Of course, if using a BVM, the operator would need to remain in the MRI room itself along with the patient. Although no adverse health effects from magnetic waves have been discovered, it is perhaps prudent to limit one's exposure. In addition, the MRI machine itself is extremely loud, almost to the point of being disorienting to anesthesia providers.

Our regular anesthesia machines and intensive care ventilators are made of iron and steel, so they are not appropriate for use in the MRI suite. At least one report from a decade ago, however, showed some ingenuity: the anesthesia machine was bolted to the inside wall of the MRI room. We, however, are not that brave—we watched too many Wile E. Coyote cartoons when we were younger. He always had bad luck with magnets and large ferromagnetic objects.

In some instances, a hole in the wall can provide entry of a long circle circuit with the anesthesia machine outside the MRI room. There are commercially available MRI compatible anesthesia machines that are able to provide manual and positive-pressure ventilation as well as inhalational agents through non-ferromagnetic vaporizers. These machines are made of aluminum and various plastics. In addition, small MRI-compatible "transport" ventilators, briefcase sized, can be used to provide positive-pressure ventilation. Ventilators such as these are pneumatically driven from a wall source of oxygen (or an aluminum cylinder).

SOURCE OF MEDICAL GASES

Imagine a heavy, full oxygen tank flying through the air into the middle of the MRI magnet "donut"; this has happened on several occasions. With some reports, a patient was in the MRI at that time, resulting in serious injury to the patient. Even if an MRI machine was empty when this happened, it remained a problem. The magnet of an MRI machine is not easily turned off, and when it is, the cost to turn one back on and the time lost in this are significant. Some facilities do not even allow standard gas cylinders in the general area of the MRI equipment, let alone in the actual MRI room.

Most MRI suites have pipeline medical gas supply if not in the actual MRI room, then within a distance that long gas hoses can be used. Those that do not will have a supply of aluminum oxygen cylinders. Flowmeters are also available for MRI use for nasal cannula, mask, or even Mapleson circuit use. Most suction canister apparatuses are safe for MRI use.

MONITORING

Conventional monitors for electrocardiography (ECG) and pulse oximetry are problematic in the MRI suite. They may contain ferromagnetic material and could become projectiles. Another problem is radiofrequency (RF) interference. RF interferes with the quality of the MRI image. The housing of MRI-compatible monitors needs to be constructed out of material that blocks leakage of RF. RF can also be responsible for heating of ECG leads and pulse oximeter probes enough to cause burns to the patient. Looped ECG leads are especially bad for this; we won't go into the physics of that, however.

To prevent excess RF and decrease the danger of burns to the patient, ECG leads are made out of insulated graphite wire. Graphite wire leads heat up less in the MRI environment than standard leads. Leads are also shorter to decrease loops of ECG wire being formed during placement and imaging. From where the leads meet coming from the patient, the cable back to the monitor box is fiberoptic instead of wire cable. The ECG pads are also made with graphite snaps or buttons to attach to the leads. Although this setup is adequate for monitoring of rhythm, it is not as good as standard leads and pads to monitor for ST-segment changes.

Pulse oximeter probes for MRI use contain a minimum of ferromagnetic material, and the cable connecting the probe to the monitor box is fiberoptic in nature.

Something to keep in mind is that even though a monitor may be MRI compatible, there are differences in MRI compatibility. Some monitors have enough ferromagnetic material in them that they are only safe for use at a certain distance from the magnet or only up to a certain magnetic force strength (measured in Teslas). There is at least one case report of an MRI-compatible monitor that was sucked into the magnet because the monitor had gotten closer than the recommended 5-foot distance.

Either the anesthesia provider can stay in the room with the patient during the MRI, or it is acceptable in such circumstances to leave and watch the patient through a window or a closed-circuit camera setup. The monitor screen can be watched in the same way.

INTRAVENOUS INFUSION PUMPS

There are MRI-compatible infusion pumps available. One alternate solution is to simply have enough intravenous (IV) extension tubing to reach the patient from a standard IV pump outside the MRI room.

CONCLUSION

Fortunately, there are few equipment concerns as far as anesthetic implications for remote locations other than the MRI suite. The main concerns are working space, protection from radiation for the clinician, availability of medical gases and suction, and ability to provide adequate care in code situations. Anesthesia in remote locations, however, is not going away and will be an increasing part of your practice. So if you do not like it now, you would be well advised to learn to love it.

CAPNOGRAPHY AND GAS MONITORING

16

KEYWORDS

- instrumentation
- gas concentrations
- infrared absorption
- mass spectrometry
- Raman scatter analysis
- monitoring methods
- gas concentrations
- oxygen
- nitrogen
- carbon dioxide
- anesthetic gases and vapors

How comfortable would you be *not* having end-tidal carbon dioxide monitoring after intubating a patient? Although we might be called on to intubate a patient in the intensive care unit (ICU) or emergency department (ED) without the benefit of capnography, we certainly rely on it in the operating room (OR). It is a standard of care for our specialty. Not only do we rely on capnography to ensure tracheal intubation, but we also are able to use the values and even the waveforms derived from capnography to diagnose and treat the patient.

Along with pulse oximetry, capnography was introduced into wide usage in anesthesia in the mid 1980s. Then clinicians had two monitors that aided in the detection of two of the most dreaded and serious events that could happen during a case: unseen hypoxemia and undetected esophageal intubation. Before capnography, undetected esophageal intubation was a main cause of anesthesia morbidity and mortality. There are old stories of the surgeon saying the blood looked darker than normal being the first symptom of esophageal intubation. What panic that would cause!

Although anesthetic agent respiratory monitoring is not as vital to good outcomes as end-tidal carbon dioxide is, it is a standard of care. We rely on it in a myriad of ways during an anesthetic case. This chapter discusses the history, types, and physics (ouch!) involved with capnography and anesthetic respiratory gas monitoring.

We will not go into the physiology and interpretation of capnography waveforms. Although it is a fascinating subject and is of importance for you to know, this topic is covered in other texts in a more detailed way than we could do here. We encourage you to learn as much as you can about capnography waveform interpretation because not only is it vital for you to know in order to provide good care to the patient, it is also often of value when you need to troubleshoot problems with your machine or monitor.

A BRIEF HISTORY

You can go into as much detail regarding the *history* of capnography as you want, much in the same way that you can go into as much detail regarding the *physics* of capnography and anesthetic gas monitoring as you want. Again, we stand on giants' shoulders; contributions from chemists, physicists, electrical engineers, and physiologists all connect into capnography. It should not be a surprise to you that much of the driving force to develop capnography in fact came from the study of respiratory physiology. The first regular clinical use of capnography was not in the OR, but in the ICU during care of ventilated patients. As mentioned, capnography became common in the OR in the mid 1980s and became an American Society of Anesthesiologists standard of care in 1991.

TYPES AND TECHNOLOGY

Three main technologies are used in clinical capnography: infrared, Raman scattering, and mass spectrometry. The first kind used clinically was the mass spectrometer. We will discuss all three of these types. In addition, capnometers can be divided into types by *where* they measure the respiratory sample: one type measures the sample in the anesthesia circuit (mainstream, or non-diverting), and the other kind takes a sample from the circuit and measures it inside a monitor (sidestream, or diverting). We will explain and discuss the pros and cons of mainstream versus sidestream sampling and then discuss the technologies used for capnography and anesthetic gas monitoring.

Types

Mainstream

This type measures carbon dioxide from within the patient's anesthesia circuit. A special attachment called a *cuvette* is placed at the Y piece. The cuvette is slightly smaller than, and looks like, a heat and moisture exchange (HME) filter. An adaptor snaps over the cuvette. The adaptor is where the electrical parts are located and has a cable that runs to the display screen. An infrared radiation (IR) generator is inside the adaptor, which shines the IR through the clear window of the cuvette to a sensor that is also built into the adaptor. Using IR spectroscopy, the carbon dioxide at the Y piece is measured in real time for each inspiration and expiration.

This is the type of capnometer that you may see in an ICU or ED. Many vital sign monitors have a module that can be used for mainstream capnography. Mainstream monitors need regular calibration by attaching the adaptor to a special calibrating cuvette that is built into the adaptor cable. Some mainstream capnometers also incorporate an oxygen analyzer. Because there is no gas siphoned out of the patient circuit with a mainstream type monitor, there is nothing to have to send to the scavenging system, such as in sidestream monitors. The cuvettes are reusable after sterilization. There are methods or attachments that allow the clinician to measure end-tidal carbon dioxide via nasal cannula with mainstream sampling. Mainstream sampling is said to be faster than sidestream sampling, but it is not so fast as to make you want to use a mainstream monitor over a sidestream type for that reason alone.

There are a few disadvantages to mainstream monitoring. Blood or secretions inside the cuvette can interfere with proper function. The cuvette/adaptor assembly is relatively heavy compared to the rest of the anesthesia circuit, and it can pull on the endotracheal tube or laryngeal mask airway, possibly kinking or dislodging the tube. It generates heat, and although it is not that warm to touch, there have been reports of the adaptor causing burns on patients when it was touching them for a prolonged period. The adaptor itself is fragile and could be put out of action if it was dropped on the floor. The authors have noticed also that the spring that helps keep the adaptor snapped onto the cuvette is easily broken, making it difficult to keep the adaptor in position.

The biggest disadvantage historically to the mainstream type of capnometer is that it did not measure any other gas or agent besides carbon dioxide (and oxygen if the system also has an oxygen analyzer). Although the measurement of only carbon dioxide and oxygen meets the standard of care, most clinicians definitely preferred to also have the ability to measure inspired and exhaled anesthetic agents. Although now there are mainstream capnometer designs that indeed measure anesthetic agents, the earlier ability of sidestream capnometry to do this made sidestream monitoring more widespread.

Sidestream

In this type, a sample of gas is diverted from the patient circuit through a small tube that comes off the circuit near or at the Y piece. This sample travels through the tubing into the monitor box itself. This is the type that is used by most current capnometers and anesthetic gas monitors. Technologies that use or used sidestream sampling include mass spectrometry, Raman spectroscopy, and infrared spectroscopy. Therefore, unlike mainstream sampling, sidestream sampling can be used by monitors capable of measuring not only end-tidal carbon dioxide but all the other anesthetic gases and agents as well.

Sidestream sampling is easily used with a nasal cannula for capnography, using either a homemade version or a specially designed monitoring cannula. The special type of cannula has the sampling line built into the cannula itself, and some have a small spoon-shaped piece of plastic that sits below the nasal prongs that funnels the exhalations of mouth breathers into the sampling line ports. You can even rig the nasal cannula to monitor through the lumen of an oral airway. If you are in the magnetic resonance imaging suite, you can simply add extra tubing to the sampling line to monitor the capnogram.

By the way, if you do not know how to fabricate a homemade capnography-capable nasal cannula, you simply stick a 14-gauge intravenous (IV) catheter into a single prong from the opposite side of the prong opening. Remove the needle and cut the catheter off flush with the prong. Then you can attach the Luer lock of the sampling line to the end of the IV catheter. The accuracy is decreased, especially in regards to fraction of inspired oxygen (FiO_2), but nevertheless this simple technique works. (Of course, don't do this with the cannula attached to the patient!)

A few minor problems are associated with sidestream monitoring, but none are horrible enough to make you not want to use this type of capnometer. One problem is the need for scavenging the gas sample when the monitor is done with it if you are using anesthetic agents. The exhaust port of the monitor can be hooked up to the scavenger system of an anesthesia machine without too much trouble. It is even possible to return the sample through different tubing back to the patient circuit. If you are using very low flow or closed-circuit inhalational anesthesia, you must factor in how much volume per minute you are losing through the sampling line. This can be anywhere usually from 100 to 150 mL/min. However, newer models only draw off 50 mL/min; these are called *microstream* units. Especially in head and neck cases, the sampling line tubing is easily kinked, interfering with monitoring. A quick trick to alleviate this is using a roll of tape as a support around the tubing. Blood, secretions, and water condensation can also block the tubing. There is a disposable water trap at the end of the sampling line right before it goes into the monitor to catch moisture. These need to be changed on occasion. Leaks in the circuit can be caused by the Luer lock on either end of the sampling line being loose or unattached. Cracks can develop in the plastic water traps that will cause either a leak or incorrect readings.

All in all, sidestream monitoring is much more versatile than mainstream monitoring, but mainstream monitoring hardware is less expensive.

Technology

Mass Spectrometry

This was the first kind of clinically used capnometer. You may have used a "mass spec" at sometime during your education such as in chemistry lab. It is a large machine that is able to weigh charged atoms and molecules based on how far they travel when ionized in a vacuum and then deflected by an electrical or magnetic charge.

Let's look at an example. You give a basketball on the floor a shove, and it rolls along the floor. It passes a box fan, blowing air into its path. You would not expect the path of the basketball to be influenced much, if at all, by the air blown by the fan. The basketball continues along its path. Now roll a tennis ball along the floor. Because the tennis ball has less mass than the basketball, it would not surprise you too much if the fan blew the tennis ball slightly off course. Next roll a ping-pong ball along the floor and in front of the fan. You would expect the ping-pong ball, because of its lower mass, to be deflected by the fan to a greater degree than either the basketball or the tennis ball.

Now if we performed this example many times for each ball and measured the distance from straight that each ball was deflected by the fan, we would have a known averaged set of values that were repeatable in our setup, and then we could estimate that a ball weighing somewhere between a tennis ball and a ping-pong ball would be deflected by the fan at an angle somewhere between our deflection angle average for those two balls.

In a mass spectrometry, the ions are the balls, the electrical or magnetic force is the fan blowing air, and the deflection of the ions will be based on their mass, just like the deflection of the three balls on the floor in front of the fan. Matter will be deflected and travel in the mass spectrometer based on its mass, and this can be measured by comparing the length of travel to known compounds. That is how a mass spectrometer can determine the identity of a certain compound—by comparing how far its component pieces travel, and then comparing that with known values.

The exact same thing happened in these early clinical capnometers. It was actually made easier because of the decreased number of substances to which the instrument would be exposed. These monitors would not be exposed to unknowns like in a chemistry lab. They would see the same things all the time—carbon dioxide, nitrogen, halothane, enflurane, isoflurane, nitrous oxide, and oxygen. (Desflurane and sevoflurane weren't in clinical use back then.) Not only would it tell what was in the sample, but it also told how much was in the sample. You knew what the end-tidal agent was, the inspired agent, the nitrogen, as well as the all-important carbon dioxide.

There was a problem with using mass spectrometers in the OR; however, they were *huge* pieces of equipment. They would not fit on top of the anesthesia machine or even in the corner. In addition, they were complicated and had a lot of down time. They were also quite expensive. So the companies that made the technology came up with a way for all the rooms in a busy OR to use the mass spectrometer.

Each room used the same mass spectrometer, located in a remote room somewhere in the OR. Sampling lines went from a local monitor (where the readout screen and control buttons were) on top of the anesthesia machine to the central mass spectrometer. About every minute or so, the data on the screen would be updated. This was quite satisfactory—do you *really* need the end-tidal isoflurane updated constantly? No, once a minute or so is fine. But what about waiting for carbon dioxide? If you're intubating someone, you surely don't want to wait a minute before it is your room's turn again to see if you are in the trachea or not! The companies also thought of this problem. In each box on top of the anesthesia machine in each room was a separate *local* infrared capnometer. That way, you didn't have to wait for your room's turn to know if you had end-tidal carbon dioxide because the carbon dioxide analysis was done right there in the room.

All of this may seem quite dated to you, and you're correct. You can still find some facilities that may not have updated their monitoring from mass spectrometry, but mass spectrometers for anesthetic clinical use are no longer produced. But at that time, from the late 1970s (when it was first used in critical care) until the early 1990s, the mass spectrometer was the best way to perform respiratory gas analysis. Many institutions used mass spectrometry into the late 1990s and early 2000s. However, recent research with the detection of end-tidal propofol used a mass spectrometer. If end-tidal propofol monitoring becomes commonplace one day, though, it is doubtful that mass spectrometry will return to clinical use because infrared monitors will be modified to measure end-tidal propofol.

Back in those days, you probably would have heard about "Sara" or "Elmer," depending on what brand of mass spec was used at your hospital. "Sara" stood for "System for Anesthetic and Respiratory Analysis," which was made by a company called PPG-Biomedical, and "Elmer" referred to "Perkin-Elmer," the manufacturer of another clinical anesthesia mass spectrometer system.

Raman Scattering

This does not have to do with spilling noodles; in the 1920s, a man named C.V. Raman discovered that when you shine light onto a compound, some of the light bounces off the molecules of that compound at a different wavelength than the original light. In addition to measuring this new wavelength, the intensity of the new wavelength that comes off the compound can be measured. When compared with a catalog of known values, you can tell what the compound is and what its concentration is. This is called Raman spectroscopy because it is based on the process of Raman scattering. Raman won the Nobel Prize in 1930 for this work.

Raman spectroscopy was adapted to clinical anesthesia in the late 1980s. It was a good system for its time. It could do all the things that a mass spectrometer system could do but in a much smaller package, right in the individual OR. The system was called "Rascal" (RAman SCattering AnALyzer). The light that was used was an argon beam laser, and about once a month or so, a small Thermos bottle–sized cylinder of argon was changed out on the back of the machine.

This technology is no longer in common use in clinical anesthesia. Infrared gas monitoring was, and is, cheaper to buy and to maintain.

Infrared Analysis

This is the most commonly used anesthetic gas monitoring system. This technology is cheaper than the previously mentioned methods, so it has more or less replaced any other means of capnography and anesthetic gas monitoring. The two previously mentioned technologies, mass spectrometry and Raman spectroscopy, are really only of historic interest. Probably every gas monitor you will now uses infrared spectroscopy.

Infrared technology relies on the fact that different substances absorb different wavelengths of light. This is also discussed in Chapter 17 on pulse oximetry. Simply put, infrared light is shined through the sample gas from the patient's airway or circuit, and based on what wavelengths of infrared light the sensor detects (meaning the infrared light that the molecules in the sample *did not* absorb), the monitor can tell the type and amount of gas or vapor present in the sample.

Infrared radiation gas monitoring systems are designed so that there are multiple chambers, so simultaneous measurements of the components of the sample are done. (The mass spectrometer and Raman scattering types also have multiple chambers.) Sample analysis is quick enough that you get inspired and expired results. They are now designed so small that they are easily portable, and may be built in to transport monitors.

The traditional type of infrared device is called "black body." The black body type generates its infrared light from a heating element inside the monitor. This type works fine, but the kind of IR that is produced in this manner is made up of many different wavelengths that are not needed, so filters are used to keep those out of the sampling chamber, allowing only the radiation that is useful for gas monitoring. Smaller units have been designed using what is called "microstream" technology, which uses IR that comes from a laser source. This cuts down on the amount of unused IR radiation that is produced. Microstream also uses far less of a sample amount per minute: 50 mL/min versus the 100 to 150 mL/min that black body units siphon from the patient circuit.

Infrared radiation technology has one main drawback: it cannot detect and measure molecules that are made up of the same atoms, such as elemental oxygen and nitrogen (O_2 and N_2). This means that another form of oxygen sensor is needed, and because nitrogen is undetectable, you cannot rely on the monitor to tell you when a large amount of nitrogen (e.g., from an air embolism) appears. The mass spectroscopy and Raman spectroscopy types did measure these two gases.

DISPOSABLE (CHEMICAL) CAPNOMETERS

Most of you have probably seen or used disposable capnometers. They are especially handy for first responders and are also commonly stocked on code carts in health care settings. They are reminiscent of an HME and have 15-mm adaptors to fit in the circuit at the Y piece or to the endotracheal tube adaptor. These devices incorporate a disk of filter paper that is impregnated with a chemical base and an indicator. The pH changes when exposed to carbon dioxide on exhalation, so the color of the filter paper changes. On inspiration, the color reverts to its initial shade. What colors are involved depend on the type chemistry and brand that is involved.

These devices are mainly good for qualitative, not quantitative, information even though there is a built-in scale from which to compare the color shades that are generated. You'll more or less find out the presence or absence of carbon dioxide and that its level is low, medium, or high. But for what they are designed for, that is good enough. However, in a true code or cardiac arrest situation, if there is very little or no carbon dioxide exchange, disposable capnometers will be of limited value because there might not be enough carbon dioxide in the exhalations to cause the color to change. They will work for quite a while, and one of the authors has even done a whole case using one when at a remote location and the regular capnometer failed. Secretions, gastric contents, and moisture are the devices'

Table 16-1 **TYPES OF ANESTHETIC GAS MONITORS**		
Type	**Advantages**	**Disadvantages**
Mass spectrometry	Earliest technology used clinically in anesthesia… Can measure anesthetic agent… Can measure elemental molecules (e.g., O_2, N_2)… Accurate…	Expensive… Not portable… No longer in clinical use… One spectrometer shared by several rooms… Slow because of shared locations…
Raman scattering	Individual monitor for each location can measure anesthetic agent… Can measure elemental molecules (e.g., O_2, N_2)… Accurate… Portable…	Need to change out argon tanks… Expensive… Higher maintenance costs… No longer in clinical use…
Infrared	Individual monitor for each location… Rapid response… Relatively inexpensive… Small and portable… Low maintenance costs…	Cannot measure elemental molecules (e.g., O_2, N_2)… Needs built-in oxygen sensor…
Chemical	Inexpensive… Highly portable… Needs no electricity… Ease of use… Accurate for presence of CO_2…	No waveform… Inaccurate quantitatively… Can be ruined by secretions or gastric contents… Color change can be difficult to see (e.g., dark room)… Color changes may be minimal to none in certain circumstances (e.g., cardiac arrest)… Measures CO_2 only…

worst enemies and interfere with proper function. Table 16-1 lists several types of gas monitors.

OXYGEN ANALYZERS

Other chapters have discussed many different ways to ensure that we do not deliver a hypoxic mixture. Here is another way. It is a regulation that an anesthesia machine has an oxygen analyzer of some sort. Some types of machines have an analyzer built into them somewhere, almost always at the inspiratory limb adaptor. Other machines that are integrated with a gas monitor rely on the monitor's detection of oxygen. Some machines have both.

There are two main ways to analyze oxygen on an anesthesia machine. Of course, mass spectrometry and Raman spectroscopy were able to give you oxygen readings, but they are not in clinical use to any degree now. One way is by electrochemical means; there are electro-galvanic sensors and polarographic electrode sensors. The other is by a paramagnetic system.

Electro-galvanic

This is the type that is usually incorporated into the anesthesia machine itself in the area of the origin of the inspiratory limb. Calibration of this analyzer is a part of the morning checkout of such a machine. These types of devices are also used in diving applications.

How does an electro-galvanic oxygen sensor work? There is a fuel cell, reminiscent of a battery, about 1 inch by 1 inch or so in size, inside the apparatus. Inside the fuel cell is potassium hydroxide. At one end of the cell is a thin lead anode, and at the other end is a gold cathode. When oxygen and potassium hydroxide meet, an electrical current is formed between the two metal electrodes that is proportional to the concentration of oxygen. This current is then read as what percent of oxygen is in the gas that the fuel cell is exposed to. These fuel cells have a limited shelf life of 6 to 12 months even when in a vacuum-sealed foil pouch. Upon exposure to air, they begin to degrade.

If you have ever calibrated one of these, you know the response is relatively slow. It is not possible for such an analyzer to give breath-to-breath inspired and expired concentrations of oxygen; it functions only to tell you how much oxygen is reaching the inspiratory limb. Of course, ideally the sensor would be located right at the Y piece as close to the patient as possible, but the weight and size of the sensor make that impractical.

Polarographic

This kind is similar to the electro-galvanic type of sensor. But instead of a fuel cell, a gas-permeable membrane is attached to a power source and an electrolyte. Oxygen diffuses through the membrane and is reduced to hydroxide ions. A current is formed during this that is proportional to the amount of oxygen present. This type of sensor is found at the takeoff of the inspiratory limb, just like the electro-galvanic sensor. The membrane and electrolyte are package together and need to be replaced when the electrolyte or the membrane is depleted.

Paramagnetic

Did you know that oxygen is attracted to a magnetic field? Oxygen is an example of a *paramagnetic* gas, and it is the only paramagnetic gas we use in anesthesia practice. This property of oxygen allows it to be measured by its reaction in a magnetic field.

In this type of analyzer, the sample you are concerned with is compared to a reference source, usually room air ($FiO_2 = 0.21$). The sample gas flows through one tube, and the reference flows through another tube; both tubes are in close proximity to an electromagnet. There is a pressure transducer located between these two tubes that measures the pressure difference from one tube to the other. The electromagnet is turned on and off rapidly, with a frequency of 100 to 160 Hz. With each pulse of the magnet, oxygen in both tubes expands toward the magnet, causing a pressure wave. The pressure transducer between the sample line and the reference line measures the pressure variations, which is turned into an electric signal that is proportional to the oxygen concentration difference between the two tubes. The readout is very rapid and is how gas monitors give you inspired and end-tidal oxygen concentrations. Remember that infrared analyzers cannot measure oxygen, so the gas monitor of your anesthesia workstation will have not only infrared spectroscopy for carbon dioxide and agent concentrations but also a separate oxygen analyzer built into it, probably of the paramagnetic variety.

CONCLUSION

We certainly hope you know more now about gas monitoring than you did before you read this chapter. We are most fortunate to be blessed with such technology that surrounds us in everything we do clinically. To be the best clinician possible, it is wise to understand the inner workings of all those boxes all around you when you give an anesthetic.

PULSE OXIMETRY | 17

KEYWORDS

- pulse oximetry
- alarms and safety features
- oxygen

Imagine performing an anesthetic without a pulse oximeter. Unless you have been an anesthesiologist or anesthetist for a very long time, you have never done a case without a pulse oximeter. In fact, if you had to have just one single monitor, you would probably choose a "pulse ox." It tells you at least three things: it tells you the patient's oxygen saturation, naturally, but it also tells you the patient's pulse, the fact that the patient's heart is beating, and that the patient has enough of a systolic blood pressure to allow the probe to pick up a signal.

But anesthetics were done for around 130 years before pulse oximetry became commonplace. It is a testament to how important and how revolutionary the pulse oximetry is that a generation or two after its introduction, none of us would *ever* do a case without one.

"Revolutionary" is a good word to use because the pulse oximeter and its colleague, the capnograph, came into common clinical practice at around the same time. Anesthetic practice received not one but two blessings in the 1980s. Both technologies quickly became standard of care. Nothing since then has come close to rivaling the benefits that these monitors give us for each and every case.

Anesthesia monitors can be divided into two groups: patient or physiologic monitors, such as a noninvasive blood pressure monitor, and safety monitors, such as an oxygen sensor. A pulse oximeter is a combination of both a physiologic monitor *and* a safety monitor. It tells us something about the physiologic status of the patient, with regard to ventilation, oxygenation, pulse, and so forth, plus it lets us know that the patient is in fact being oxygenated or not. Remember, the delivery of oxygen is the main function of an anesthesia machine, in our minds, as we discussed earlier in this book.

PHYSICS

Physics, although perhaps having a reputation among those of us who majored in biology, zoology, and so forth in college as being hard and boring, is really just the study of how things work. Therefore, to understand how something works, you have to talk about physics at least a *little* bit. Again, you can go into the physics of pulse oximetry as deeply as you desire, but in this discussion, we will only discuss the physics of pulse oximetry that we think is important for you to know.

When you were a kid, you probably played with a flashlight by holding your hand over the beam and seeing how the light made your hand look. Some of the light was absorbed by your hand because the beam was not as bright leaving your hand as it was entering your hand. A pulse oximeter shines light through your hand (or wherever you have attached the probe) and measures how much light comes out the other side.

Pulse oximetry works because of the differences in the type and amount of light that oxygenated and deoxygenated hemoglobin absorb, respectively. The pulse oximetry probe shines two LED lights through the vascular bed. One light is red, at a wavelength of 660 nanometers (nm), and the other is an infrared beam of 940 nm of wavelength. The red light is absorbed by reduced hemoglobin more than oxygenated hemoglobin. Conversely, the infrared light is absorbed by oxygenated hemoglobin more than reduced hemoglobin.

The other side of the probe is the sensor, or photodiode. It picks up the amount of red and infrared light that *was not* absorbed by the reduced and oxygenated hemoglobin. Software in the monitor itself takes the data received and translates it into a number and a waveform for us.

But remember that it is called a *pulse* oximeter, not just an oximeter. The pulse is very important to obtaining a reading. It is the pulse that enables the sensor to distinguish between arterial blood and capillary or venous blood in the bed being monitored. The LED lights flash at 100 times a second. You can almost believe that you can make out the flashing if you look at a probe, but in reality, that would be hard. Think of it—a cartoon shows still pictures at 24 frames a second, and it looks seamless. But it is the flashing, pulsating light that allows the oximeter to detect the pulse of arterial blood in the monitored bed. It measures the high and low readings, and the difference is the pulse of arterial blood.

All of this goes back to what is called Beer's law, or the Beer-Lambert law. It is a way of analyzing substances by light absorption. It is also called spectrophotometry. Those of you who majored or minored in chemistry probably in one exercise had an unknown substance and you had to figure out what it was by using spectrophotometry. We will definitely *not* go into depth on Beer's law except to refresh your memories from college chemistry and remind you that it has to do with identifying substances based on their absorption of light. Beer's law is also mentioned in the chapter on capnography.

SYSTEM DESIGN

Initially, when pulse oximetry was introduced into anesthetic practice, the monitors were stand-alone units. Stand-alone units are still available, but most of the time now, the oximeter is integrated into a combination monitor, with one screen on the anesthesia machine displaying all patient data. Even small transport monitors have built-in pulse oximeters. Many oximeters now are very small, the size of cell phones or even smaller. Also, most probes and cables are incompatible with equipment from other manufacturers, and the software that derives the saturation value differs from manufacturer to manufacturer.

One of the great features of pulse oximetry is the audible tone that changes with changes in SpO_2 (oxygen saturation). Nothing gets the attention of everyone in the operating room (OR)—yes, even surgeons—than the sound of a pulse oximetry getting lower and lower. The sound change with degree of oxygenation allows the operator to focus on the patient during a situation without having to continuously check the screen readout. Pulse oximeters have the ability to be programmed to the high and low alarm setting that the clinician desires. Most of us don't worry about an SpO_2 being too high, but in neonates, too much oxygen can be a bad thing.

SQI stands for "signal quality indicator" and is a measure of how good the oximeter software thinks the signal from the probe is. The different manufacturers will show the SQI of a waveform by various means, either a bar graph or a number in real time along with the pulse oximetry reading.

CLINICAL ASPECTS

Probes

Probes are either of the disposable, one-time-use variety, or reusable. The disposable types come in different sizes for pediatric through adult use and in different shapes and configurations for use at various sites. They mostly consist of the LED lights, sensor, and wiring to connect to the cable and are covered in tape to stick on the site you place it. The reusable types are generally more robustly made for repeated use and are of a "clothes pin" or finger sleeve configuration. These days, disposable probes are very common, especially in light of following contact precautions. The next patient cannot be contaminated by using the same probe. Inpatients keep their disposable probes on for days, and they are used not only in the ORs but also in postanesthesia care units, critical care units, and monitored floor beds and during transport. In the past, disposable probes were reused frequently from patient to patient with varying results. Wiring would fray, and tape needed to be reinforced to keep the probe on the patient's finger. Some companies, however, take used disposable probes and repackage them after checking their function and cleaning them.

Monitoring Sites

Multiple sites for probe placement have been documented and used. Anywhere where you can place a probe is fair game. Of course, the most commonly used site is a finger. We prefer to place the probe on the fifth "pinky" finger; patients often rub their eyes after emergence, and a bulky, stiff-cornered probe on the second or third finger can lead to a corneal abrasion.

Other obvious sites are the toes and earlobes. Thenar and hypothenar eminences can be used. The palms and feet can be used for pediatric patients. Sites that are less commonly used include the nose and forehead (specially shaped probes are available for these sites), web spaces, penis, tongue, and cheek. For the tongue and cheek (buccal) sites, the nose wire from an OR facemask (the kind you wear, not the kind you put on the patient) can be taped to the exterior side of a disposable probe to give it a "backbone" and permanent shape to better approximate the lights and sensor. One report described taping a disposable probe with LEDs and sensor exposed to an oral airway.

We commonly place buccal probes on burn patients, on whom there may not be anywhere else to place a probe, and on trauma patients. The facial artery is a branch of the carotid system and maintains its pulse better than digits during a state of hypovolemia, hypotension, and decreased perfusion.

| PROBLEMS

No system is foolproof. It is possible to obtain false-positive and false-negative data from pulse oximetry. In fact, because of wishful thinking, we like to believe that all low readings are spurious. That is true sometimes but does not mean that low readings simply can be assumed to be false-negative results. Matters still should be investigated. Interestingly enough, we never worry about false-positive pulse oximeter values, do we?

Things that can cause problems with accurate signals include, but are not limited to, patient movement, hypothermia, hypovolemia, shock, improper placement of probe (in which it is coming off or that the LED light doesn't line up on a path directly into the photodiode sensor), paint, fingernail polish (but not red or pink colors usually), artificial fingernails, and extraneous light (OR and ceiling lights). A good trick to decrease the problem with lights is to wrap the finger and probe in the foil pack that an alcohol swab comes in.

In the case of methemoglobinemia, the pulse oximeter value will decrease until it reaches a level of 85%, and it stays there. With carboxyhemoglobinemia, the carboxyhemoglobin has a similar light absorption pattern to oxygenated hemoglobin, so the readings given by the monitor will be falsely high. Some injected dyes, mainly methylene blue, interfere with the pulse oximetry reading for 5 minutes or so after injection.

It is important for any anesthesia practitioner to realize that pulse oximetry is not a reliable indicator of successful endotracheal intubation. But it is true that if you intubate a severely cyanotic patient and the SpO_2 improves you are likely in the trachea. But if you have a patient who you have preoxygenated for several minutes before induction, the saturation could stay high for a couple of minutes after you have intubated the esophagus. Pulse oximetry is not a substitute for capnography.

We used the term "revolutionary" when we began this chapter in describing the effect that the introduction of pulse oximetry had on the practice of anesthesiology. That is true, but what you might not know is there has never been a study that thoroughly proves that pulse oximetry improves morbidity and mortality. A study in 1993 showed that although pulse oximetry allowed clinicians to detect hypoxemia more quickly, there was no significant change in patient outcomes. That being said, pulse oximetry nevertheless became a standard of care long *before* this study was published. Studies showed that clinicians felt more comfortable when they monitored SpO_2 on patients, so despite the lack of evidence that pulse oximeters improved overall outcomes, they were in the OR to stay. Nobody wanted to give up that monitoring ability. If you were practicing back then, you wouldn't have wanted to give up pulse oximetry either.

CONCLUSION

One theme of this book has been that we stand on the shoulders of giants. Johann Lambert died in 1777, and August Beer died in 1863. They had the science worked out but needed for the technology to catch up to them. Everything we do and use in anesthesia comes from the minds of very smart, dedicated people. Some are famous, but most are not. We are very blessed by their efforts.

HEMODYNAMIC MONITORING | 18

KEYWORDS

- pressure transducers: resonance
- damping
- noninvasive blood pressure measurement
- oscillometry

The frequent measurement of a patient's arterial blood pressure (BP) is *standard care* in anesthesia. The guidelines state that BP must be measured, but *how* it is measured is up to you. Is the presence of a pulse an indicator of adequate BP? No, not really. But that was how it was done in the distant past. In some modern situations, however, a finger on a pulse is all you may have to work with until help comes. Is a sphygmomanometer an acceptable way to monitor BP? Yes, it is, if the operator is capable of reliably using one. The problem with sphygmomanometers is that they are labor intensive. But up until the mid 1980s, that is just how most BPs were taken when a patient was under an anesthetic.

Fortunately for us, there are now ways to measure BP that require less work on our part. Noninvasive BP monitoring (NIBP) relies on an oscillometer to give us an accurate BP reading. All we have to do is place the BP cuff on the patient, press "start," and tell the monitor how often we want it to measure BP. The other method of measuring BP is with an intraarterial catheter. This is an example of *invasive monitoring* versus the other ways we mentioned, which are classed as *noninvasive monitoring*.

Of course, the kind of BP monitoring is chosen for use in an anesthetic is a complicated subject. Much of the decision depends on the kind of case and the physical status of the patient. But we will not get into that here. We want you to understand how both invasive and noninvasive BP monitoring works.

INVASIVE BLOOD PRESSURE MONITORING

Depending on the rotation you are on or the type of patient you anesthetize regularly, you may use a pressure transducer every day. Invasive BP monitoring, central venous pressure (CVP) measurements, and pulmonary artery catheter readings all require a transducer somewhere between the patient and the monitor display. (Okay, you could use a columnar manometer, but that would be really inconvenient.)

You can go into as much physics with pressure monitoring and transducers as you want. It would take an electrical engineer or physicist to understand pressure transducers inside and out. Don't worry; we aren't engineers or physicists either. So if we can understand it, so can you. The bottom line is that we use these things very frequently, but we have no idea how they work. Yes, it *is* complicated, but we will try to make it as simple as possible so we all can understand this extremely important but underappreciated marvel. But we *will* have to talk about some physics to get to where we want to go.

Parts of a Transducer

You can divide a transducer into two main parts, the patient connection and the electrical system. The patient side includes everything from the catheter inside the patient to the transducer diaphragm, and the electrical system is everything from the diaphragm to the monitor. The diaphragm is inside the plastic part where the connector cable and the flush device are. As you may guess, when all this technology hit the operating room (OR) from the physics lab several decades ago, the transducer was *not* disposable. Now, of course, they are, and it would be interesting to know how many transducers are wasted each year because a resident decided an arterial line or a CVP would be a good idea but his or her attending said, "No, I think we'll be okay without one." We will talk first about the physics and different parts of the electrical system of the transducer and then the physics and parts of the patient-to-transducer part of the system.

Physics of the Transducer–Electrical System

In simple terms, a transducer takes one kind of energy and changes it into another kind of energy. In our case, a transducer takes mechanical energy (hydrostatic pressure) and changes it into electrical energy. The transducers we use in the OR are a type of *strain gauge*. A strain gauge has a diaphragm that oscillates with each pressure waveform, and this movement changes the resistance in a resistor that is part of a *Wheatstone bridge*.

Now we're really getting deep into physics. The Wheatstone bridge was originally invented by a man named Samuel Christie in 1833 but was improved by Charles Wheatstone in 1843. (Somehow Christie was unlucky as far as the eponym. But don't blame Wheatstone; he still called his improvement the Christie bridge, but everyone else started calling it the Wheatstone bridge.)

Back to physics; the Wheatstone bridge is shaped like a four-sided diamond, and each side has a resistor on it. There are two resistors of a known resistance, one resistor that can be made to vary in its amount of resistance and one of an unknown resistance. There is also a source of electricity attached, allowing current to flow through the bridge, because the purpose is to balance both halves of the diamond, so that the sum of resistors 1 and 2 equals the resistance of the variable and the unknown resistor. It is *that* resistor with the unknown resistance that is attached to our strain gauge diaphragm.

There is also a *galvanometer* (something that measures amount and direction of electric flow) that measures the direction of electrical flow between the two sides of the diamond. When the flow is balanced, or a net flow of zero, the resistance of the unknown side of the diamond is known. That is the side, remember, that is attached to our strain gauge, and it is that resistance that is proportional to our pressure we are measuring by our strain gauge. The diagram in Figure 18-1 will help.

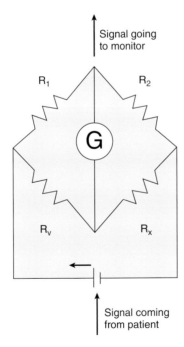

Figure 18-1 ▪ Schematic of a Wheatstone bridge. The value of resistors R_1 and R_2 are known. R_x is the unknown resistance caused by the action of the pressure waveform on the transducer diaphragm. R_v is a resistor whose resistance is varied until there is no net flow through the galvanometer, G. When R_1 R_2 is equal to R_v R_x, the bridge is balanced, and the resistance value is converted into a hemodynamic pressure value by the monitor.

The important thing to remember is that the transducer changes the pressure that we are measuring in the patient (arterial, CVP, and so on) and changes it into electrical energy that is read by our monitor by use of measuring resistance through a Wheatstone bridge.

The electrical adaptor of the transducer attaches to a cable that goes to our monitoring system either directly or through a shelf of "boxes" that is ultimately attached to the monitor. There is an amplifier that increases the intensity of the reading coming from the transducer, and then there is various hardware and software that gives us the nice tracing with numbers that we see on the screen.

So now we're all done with the physics part of this chapter, right? We are sorry, but no. We need to discuss the physics of the patient part of the transducer, too.

Physics of the Transducer–Patient Connection

At first, it might not seem that there is any physics relating to the section of the pressure transducer between the patient's vascular system and the electrical stuff. But there is, and the physics of the patient connection involves things that *we* can control.

Damping and Underdamping

The physics of the patient side of the transducer has to do with the concept of damping, its counterpart underdamping, and the resonance of the system. These concepts are often seen on keyword lists, and you are expected to know about them for your board examinations.

Damping (sometimes called *overdamping*) is a term that relates to anything that decreases the quality or intensity of the pressure waveform energy before it gets to the transducer diaphragm. *Underdamping* is a term that relates to anything that exaggerates the quality or intensity of the pressure waveform on its way to the transducer. There are more things that cause damping (or overdamping) than things that cause underdamping. We will discuss damping and underdamping as they relate to each part or factor of the patient side of the transducer.

Tubing   The initial thing you may have noticed when you were hooking up your first art line was that the tubing is different than regular IV tubing. Because it is different, there must be a reason it is different, right?

Pressure transducers come with *high-pressure* tubing. The tubing is thicker, stiffer, and less compliant than an intravenous (IV) setup. This is because regular IV tubing would interfere with accurate pressure readings because it would *absorb* some of the energy of the pressure waveform and cause *damping* of the waveform. The waveform that was generated would be less in intensity, especially for the higher or systolic value. This wouldn't be too much of a problem if measuring CVP, but it would be a problem for pulmonary artery pressure monitoring and especially systemic arterial monitoring.

Tubing Length The length of tubing for a transducer as it comes out of the package is around 4 feet. That length is long enough to reach from the catheter site to where you have placed the transducer. Although the length is not written in stone, it is a compromise between having enough tubing to work with but not enough to cause significant damping. We all have probably had to add high-pressure extension tubing to a transducer setup to meet our needs in the OR, but you should remember that additional tubing length causes damping even if you use high-pressure tubing. Likewise, less tubing than normal can cause underdamping.

Tubing length affects damping in two ways. The first way is that with excess tubing, there is more surface area of tubing to absorb the waveform traveling inside it. Second, more tubing increases the mass of fluid that the waveform must move in order to propagate its energy to the transducer diaphragm. Both of these contribute to damping of the waveform.

Fluid Path The fluid path is the medium in which the waveform energy travels. Fluid is relatively incompressible compared with air. As an example, fill a 10-cc syringe with air and attach it to a closed stopcock. You will be able to push down on the plunger to a certain degree, compressing the air (gas) inside it. Try again with the syringe full of saline instead of air. You will not be able to compress the plunger at all.

In a similar fashion, bubbles of air in the fluid path will be compressed by the waveform energy traveling through the fluid. Even though it seems like this loss of energy would be so small as to not influence the pressure reading, it is enough to cause damping of the waveform even when there are very small bubbles present. Conversely, if a transducer system is underdamped, an old trick was to place a small amount of air in the line to purposely dampen the waveform. It was a potentially dangerous practice, however, because if you flushed the line without removing the bubble, it would go right into the patient.

Viscosity of the fluid itself affects accuracy of the waveform. The preferred fluid for transducers is normal saline (heparinized or not). An increase in fluid path viscosity, like in an unflushed line full of blood, will dampen the waveform tracing. Although blood versus saline in a line probably will not make a significant clinical difference, blood left in a line can form a clot, usually in the catheter itself or at the tip of the catheter, which certainly will dampen the waveform.

To guard against clot formation, transducer kits are made so that when the IV bag is placed under pressure, a small amount of IV fluid infuses into the catheter each hour. This amount is around 3 cc/hr. It is important to remember to make sure the IV bag is under pressure or the catheter will clot. It is also important, like when anytime you place a bag under pressure, that you take all of the air out of the bag. If the bag or drip chamber to be upside down when you flushed the system, air could be introduced, not just into the tubing but potentially into the patient, which is a bad thing, of course.

Flushing System Every transducer comes with some form of flushing system. Some may be similar to a button that is pressed, and some may be a "pigtail" that is pulled to open the flushing system from the pressurized IV bag. Care must be taken when flushing. Our inclination is to flush until we see the line clear all the way into the patient. However, this is not a good idea. There are cases of retrograde arterial line flow from prolonged flushing. The flush goes proximally back into central circulation. For instance, if you have a radial arterial line and flush too vigorously, the flush fluid can travel up the arm, into the aortic arch, and then perhaps up the carotids to the brain. This is a bad thing, especially if there is a tiny bubble or clot traveling along with the flush. When you flush a transducer, you should flush for only a second or so, repeatedly, until the line is clear. It is believed that a short flush will not travel in a retrograde direction long enough to reach the central circulation.

Frequency Things have a *natural frequency*. You may have heard that soldiers are supposed to walk, not march, over bridges so the frequency of the synchronized footsteps will not approach the natural frequency of the bridge. If the soldiers were marching in step, the bridge would begin to sway in rhythm to the steps and could possibly collapse. If you have ever gone over a swinging footbridge, you probably know what we mean. The more forcefully you step, the more the bridge swings and sways, and if you kept stomping as you walked, it would be hard to keep standing because the bridge would be moving so much.

If you drop a tennis ball on the floor, it will bounce several times before coming to rest. In addition, each bounce will not be as high as the preceding one. We can say that the natural frequency of the tennis ball in this case is how quickly the ball bounces. Another concept in this example is the *damping coefficient*, which has to do with how quickly the ball comes to rest. We will discuss natural frequency to an extent here, but if you want to learn more about the damping coefficient, get out your old physics textbook and turn to the classical mechanics section.

Transducers also have a natural frequency. It is supposed to be any-where from 10 to 15 Hertz (Hz). You would think that frequency of the patient's intravascular waveform will correspond to whatever the heart rate is; 60 beats/min would be 1 Hz, 90 beats/min would be 1.5 Hz, 120 beats/min would be 2 Hz, and so forth. But that is not really the case because the waveform is not a true simple sine wave. Rather, the waveform itself is a combination of more than one sine wave. That is why it looks the way it does; for instance, the dicrotic notch is one sine wave added to the systolic sine wave and so on, so we get the waveform shape we are used to seeing.

These different component waves have their own frequencies. This is why sometimes you see "ringing," or an exaggerated systolic component of an arterial waveform. Such exaggerations of the systolic or diastolic curve influence what the monitor reads out as being the systolic or diastolic pressure; it will overestimate both systolic and diastolic pressures if there is too much ringing.

So how can one tell if your transducer system is too sensitive? One way is called a *fast flush*, or *step* test. You pull the flush for a second or so and make a square wave on your screen. Then release the flush quickly and see how quickly and smoothly the waveform goes back to normal. If a system is dampened, the waveform will not return to the zero line and will take its time going down. If it is underdamped, the waveform will not only return to zero, but also overshoot zero and show extra squiggles as the waveform calms back down again. If the system is okay, after you release the flush, the waveform will go back to or go slightly past zero quickly and show four or five squiggles before it calms down.

It is possible to calculate the natural frequency (f_n) of your transducer setup. You record a paper strip of your waveform tracing and then divide the paper speed by the distance between oscillations after the fast flush.

$$F_n \text{ (in Hz)} = \text{Paper speed (in mm/sec)/Distance between waveform cycles (in mm)}$$

Although this is the correct and proper procedure, who really has time to do this during a case? In our opinion, it is better to learn the three general response patterns (normal, overdamped, and underdamped) by morphology and compare mentally with the fast flush arterial line result when performing an anesthetic with an arterial line (Figure 18-2).

It may be worth for you to experiment with an arterial line if you have one during a long, stable procedure. You can add or take away extension tubing, use regular tubing instead of pressure tubing, or add a small bubble to the system (<0.5 mL, but remove it before you flush the system and don't do this with pediatric patients or patients with known right-to-left shunts). Then compare the results of a fast flush test with your original tracing.

Zeroing One of the things we always do when we hook up a transducer is to "zero" it. But exactly what does that mean? What are we "zeroing" the

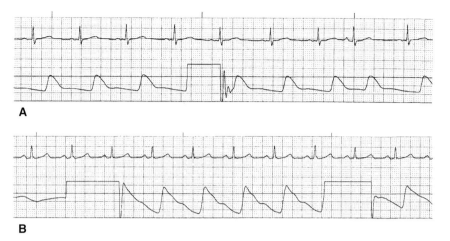

Figure 18-2 ■ (**A**) Normal response to a rapid flush test. (**B**) An overdamped waveform.

transducer to? Are we zeroing the transducer to the patient? Or to the pressure we want to measure? Or are we zeroing the transducer to the patient's position?

None of these are correct. What we are zeroing the transducer to is to *atmospheric pressure.* Why do we need to zero the transducer to atmospheric pressure? For one thing, most monitors will not give you a numerical readout without the transducer being zeroed first. You could estimate pressures based on the background scale of the monitor readout, but that would be relatively inaccurate. The other reason is that we zero the transducer to take atmospheric pressure out of the equation. What do we mean by that?

Atmospheric pressure is 760 mm Hg at sea level. If you were at sea level and your BP was 120/70 mm Hg, your actual BP would be 760 + 120/760 + 70. The atmosphere pushes in on you, and that pressure is transmitted into your body, including your vasculature. Of course, the BP cuff gauge was manufactured to take that into consideration. That is exactly what we are doing when we zero a transducer. We take into consideration whatever the atmospheric pressure is and focus on the BP, CVP, or whatever we are measuring *minus* the atmospheric pressure.

When you zero a transducer, you open the tubing up to the atmosphere at a stopcock, so the diaphragm reads atmospheric pressure; the electronics of the monitor allow you to set that pressure as *zero* on your scale.

Be mindful of *transducer drift*, also called *zero drift*. Just because you zeroed the transducer before the start of a case does not mean the transducer will remain accurate. We have seen drifts of up to −30 mm Hg, which means we were grossly undermeasuring systolic BP. It is the practice of many clinicians to rezero their transducers before coming off cardiopulmonary bypass.

You should do it really whenever you think of it. You don't need to go through the entire button-pushing procedure to do it; simply open the transducer up to air and see if the straight line goes to the zero line on the monitor scale.

NONINVASIVE BLOOD PRESSURE MONITORING

Can you imagine having to manually perform every BP measurement during an anesthetic? Well, that's how it used to be. Until automated BP monitoring became commonplace in the mid 1980s, you had to inflate the BP cuff yourself, look at a gauge, and listen for when the Korotkoff sounds came and went. Every time. At least you didn't have to hold the stethoscope on the patient's arm; there were cuffs with special stethoscope diaphragms that stayed in place for you. You had a single earpiece (the same one you used with the esophageal stethoscope discussed earlier) usually custom made to fit your ear with tubing running to the cuff diaphragm. The sphygmomanometer gauge was often built in to the anesthesia machine for easy viewing. Nevertheless, try to picture doing a complicated case or trauma and having to check the BP each time manually while hanging blood, starting lines and infusions, and so forth.

Automated NIBP has eased the work of anesthetizing. In fact, we take it for granted. Many of us have not taken a manual BP since medical or nursing school. We are used to hearing the cuff being filled with air and the sound of air being released in small amounts during the cycling process. It is almost a reassuring sound to us. But how does NIBP work? There are similarities with manual, auscultatory BP monitoring but also differences.

Noninvasive BP monitors are an example of an *oscillometer*. During the measurement cycle, the monitor picks up oscillations in the BP cuff caused by the arterial pulse and transmits them to the monitor. When the oscillations increase in amplitude, it is the systolic pressure. The oscillations continue to build in amplitude and at the maximum is mean pressure. At the point where the oscillations even out from the curve is the diastolic pressure. The oscillations are really nothing that we can pick up on, and the calculations are all done by the monitor, based on algorithms from the manufacturer (Figure 18-3).

There are a few potential problems and hazards associated with NIBP. The quickest time cycle for most units is 1 minute even though most will have a "STAT" mode that will take measurements rapidly for a couple of minutes before reverting back to its original set time cycle. Therefore, if beat-to-beat BP measurement is important for a situation, an intraarterial line would be better.

Values can be wrong with severe hypotension, as well as severe hypertension. Values are influenced by incorrect cuff sizes. A cuff too small for the patient will give a falsely increased pressure, and a cuff too small can give a falsely low pressure. A good way to remember whether the too small or too

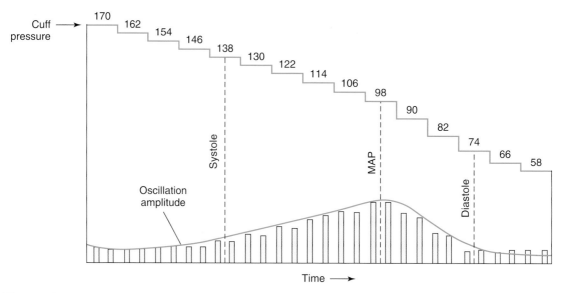

Figure 18-3 ▪ Oscillometric determination of blood pressure. (Reproduced with permission from Morgan GE, Mikhail MS, Murray MJ. *Clinical Anesthesiology.* 4th ed. New York, NY: McGraw-Hill; 2006. Table 6-5.)

large cuff causes falsely higher or lower BPs is that if you had on shoes too small for your feet, it would hurt and raise your own BP.

Also remember that the BP value that is generated is the *pressure at that time in that extremity*. If you are anesthetizing a patient in a beach chair or reverse Trendelenburg position and the cuff is on the leg, the BP in the brain is less than what the pressure in the leg is.

It can be difficult to find a good place to place the cuff on morbidly obese patients because you are trying to wrap a cylindrical shape (the cuff) around a conical shape (the arm of the obese patient). We have all had problems finding a place to put the cuff on patients with extremity injuries, previous breast surgeries, and so forth. Remember it is possible to use a neonatal-sized cuff on a finger or toe of that is the only option.

Finally, there have been instances of nerve damage and compartment syndrome on extremities on which an NIBP cuff had been used.

ACCURACY

What will be more accurate, an arterial line pressure measurement or an NIBP measurement? In truth, we probably have a tendency to believe the one that gives us the value we want. Whereas invasive direct arterial pressure monitoring can give us beat-to-beat values, an NIBP measurement is a few seconds old when the monitor displays the reading, and the BP could have changed while we were waiting on the NIBP to finish its cycle.

In either invasive or NIBP systems, the pressure value that will be the most accurate is the *mean pressure*. Remember that in invasive pressure monitoring, damping and underdamping can affect the values of systolic and diastolic pressures. Zero drift can occur. Transducer height will influence values. We all have had to readjust transducer heights when we move the OR table in some fashion. So do not blindly think that invasive arterial line pressure is accurate. If the values of BP do not make sense to you, investigate. The same goes for NIBP measurements. Incorrect cuff size, slippage of the cuff from the proper place on the extremity, and so forth can give false readings.

CONCLUSION

It is our hope that this chapter has demystified the workings of transducers and noninvasive BP monitors. This is another example of how we stand on the shoulders of giants in our daily practice; Christie and Wheatstone could not have imagined how their electric bridge could have had such a positive effect on the treatment of sick and injured patients. But we use their contributions and the contributions of countless thousands of scientists and engineers daily, not only in ORs but in all aspects of our lives. Think about all that goes into measuring pressure with a transducer—someone had to come up with how to make plastic; how to shape plastic; how to make thin, hollow needles; how to make thin catheters to slide off those thin needles; how to make monitors and software to do the things we need them to do dependably; and so on to get us to the place where we can measure BP from an arterial line. The same applies to those who made oscillometry something that could be used with an inflatable cuff around a patient's arm to give us a BP reading just by pressing a button. Every day in the OR and intensive care unit, we stand on the shoulders of giants.

BAG VALVE MASK AND MAPLESON CIRCUITS 19

KEYWORDS

- portable ventilation devices
- nonrebreathing valves
- noncircle systems

BAG VALVE MASK

The bag valve mask (BVM) is known by many different names, including manual resuscitator, self-inflating bag, and so on. It is, however, best known as an Ambu bag. Ambu is the company that introduced the BVM in the 1950s. In this discussion, the device will be referred to as a BVM.

The BVM is elegantly simple in its design. There are no parts made from metal (usually), no screws, no washers, and no springs (usually) or anything else of a complicated nature. The main parts are a self-inflating bag, with two valves (one on either end of the football-shaped and -sized bag), an inlet for fresh gas, and an outlet that both ventilates the patient and allows that ventilation to be expired.

The BVM is an unsung hero in medical care. Think of all the patients worldwide who are ventilated by a BVM at some time during the day. BVMs are used by first responders, by critical care personnel, and by anesthesia personnel. Transporting critically ill patients would be much more difficult and cumbersome without BVMs.

Bag valve masks can be used in the field, the battlefield, an ambulance, a helicopter, the emergency department, the intensive care unit, and the operating room. During disasters, BVMs may be the only type of ventilator that can work because they do not require electricity. (To be complete, there are mechanical, pneumatically powered ventilators available that do not use electricity to function, but there probably aren't that many of them in your facility, so if a disaster struck, most patients needing ventilation would be ventilated with a BVM if electrical power was interrupted.)

For anesthesia providers, the BVM also has one other important purpose: it is your spare anesthesia machine, conveniently located in a bag on your supply cart. You should never start a case, unless it is a dire emergency, without making sure you have your backup anesthesia machine in the room. Ensuring that a BVM is present should be a part of your morning checkout.

Bag Inlet Valve and Oxygen Delivery

At the end that attaches to the oxygen source (which will be called the proximal end), there is a standard clear oxygen tubing that connects to the oxygen source. This tubing is permanently joined to the proximal end of the bag. The oxygen enters the bag through a thin disc valve (bag inlet valve), which is opened by the negative pressure of the expanding self-inflating bag, as well as the pressure and flow of the oxygen from the source (Figure 19-1).

The disc valve is what keeps the contents of the self-inflating bag from leaking out the proximal end of the bag when the bag is squeezed during ventilation. The pressure of the operator's hand closes the disc valve back against its seating, closing the bag inlet valve.

So what happens to the oxygen flow during ventilation when the bag is squeezed? No oxygen can enter the bag because the bag inlet valve has closed plus the bag is being compressed anyway. That seems like a lot of gas flow to simply halt. The pressure of oxygen inside its tubing would increase and pop

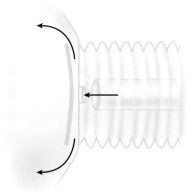

Figure 19-1 ■ Disc valve at the proximal end of the bag valve mask. Oxygen flows through coaxial inner tubing, and on self-inflation of bag, the disc valve opens, allowing filling of the bag with oxygen.

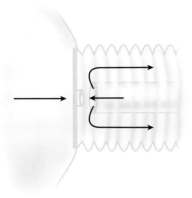

Figure 19-2 ▪ When bag is squeezed, the disc valve closes. Oxygen flow from the flowmeter continues and fills the corrugated reservoir tubing.

the connector off of the flowmeter or the increased pressure on both sides of the bag inlet valve would cause it to fail. Fortunately, there is a way for all the oxygen flow to be vented whenever the bag is squeezed.

At the place where the oxygen tubing enters the proximal end of the bag, there is a chamber that communicates with the oxygen tubing inlet. When the bag inlet valve is activated by someone squeezing the bag, the oxygen flow (which has not stopped) is vented out this opening. The oxygen coming from the flowmeter goes into a reservoir. The reservoir, in most cases, is a length of corrugated tubing coaxially situated with the oxygen tubing. It is open to the atmosphere, where excess oxygen and pressure are vented out the open end of the corrugated tubing.

This is important to understand because this topic will be revisited later on in the chapter. To reiterate, when the self-inflating bag is squeezed by the operator, the bag inlet valve closes off the oxygen delivery to the bag. This flow of oxygen is vented into the open corrugated tubing, which runs coaxially to the oxygen delivery tube. This reservoir of oxygen is used to increase the fraction of inspired oxygen (FiO_2), which is discussed later (Figure 19-2).

Self-Inflating Bag

There is really not much to say about the bag. It has two openings, one proximal and one distal. It is molded in such a way that when compressed, it rapidly returns to its normal state. The bag is textured so it is easier to grasp. Although it is not too important for anesthesiologists, the bags are made so that they can be compressed effectively while in conditions where extremes in temperatures

Table 19-1 **BAG VALVE MASK VOLUME**		
Adult	Pediatric	Neonatal
1500–2000 mL	800–1000 mL	300–500 mL

could be seen, very hot or very cold, like a first responder would encounter. The bag, and the whole apparatus for that matter, is latex free in most cases.

The average volumes for the different sizes are 1500 to 2000 mL for an adult bag, 800 to 1000 mL for a pediatric bag, and 300 to 500 mL for a neonatal bag. (However, actual tidal volumes that can be generated are much lower than these numbers; more on that later.) The bag is filled by a combination of oxygen from the flowmeter and what is in the reservoir tubing (Table 19-1).

Keep in mind, however, that many clinicians prefer to use a different kind of portable manual ventilator device when taking care of neonates and small infants (e.g., weighing <10 kg). This device is called a Jackson Rees circuit. We will discuss this circuit and the class of circuits known as the Mapleson classification later in this chapter.

Nonrebreathing Valve

The distal end, which interfaces with the patient by facemask, endotracheal (ET) tube, or supraglottic device, is called the *nonrebreathing valve*. It controls both inspiration and expiration. It is housed in a clear plastic housing, so the valve can be inspected for proper movement.

The housing itself is made with a standard-sized connector, which has a 15-mm internal diameter (for ET tubes and supraglottic devices) and 22-mm external diameter (for anesthesia facemasks).

There have been many different designs of nonrebreathing valves in the past. Many have had spring-loaded moving parts and rigid and flexible flaps. Readers are encouraged to refer to Dorsch and Dorsch for an excellent description of these kinds of valves.

The valve that will be discussed here is the fishmouth-flap nonrebreathing valve (Figure 19-3). It is really two valves in one, the fishmouth valve and the flap valve, but it is molded as one piece. The fishmouth part is what opens to ventilate the patient. It is easily seen when you look into the end of the device, right where you attach the mask or ET tube. The fishmouth sits in the middle of a soft plastic circular disc flap. The disc flap sits on its own valve seat, and when the bag is squeezed, the disc flap closes the expiration port. On expiration, when the operator stops squeezing the bag, the fishmouth closes, the circular flap relaxes off its valve seat, and passive expiration occurs.

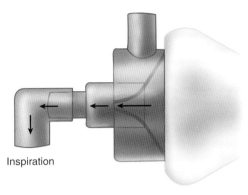

Inspiration

Figure 19-3 ▪ Nonrebreathing valve at the distal end of a bag valve mask. When the bag is squeezed to initiate positive-pressure ventilation, the flat disc section of the fishmouth valve is pushed onto its seat, and the fishmouth opens, allowing ventilation of patient through the fishmouth.

The external port, where the exhalation is exhausted into the atmosphere, is also part of the clear plastic housing of the nonrebreathing valve assembly. As mentioned, when the bag is squeezed, the disc flap of the fishmouth-flap valve closes the expiratory port, and when the flap relaxes off its seating, the expiratory port is opened (Figure 19-4). Manufacturers purposely design the exhalation port to not be the same size as the inspiratory connector and

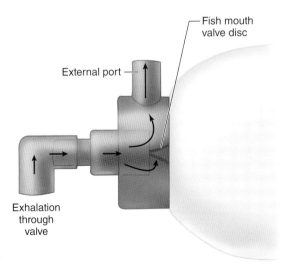

Fish mouth valve disc

External port

Exhalation through valve

Figure 19-4 ▪ Exhalation through a nonrebreathing valve. When the self-inflating bag refills, the disc comes off of its seat, and exhalation from the patient passes around it to the external port.

put ridges inside the external port opening so the mask or ET tube cannot be placed there by mistake.

Some external ports come with a caplike deflector, which can direct the exhalation away from the operator. It is easily removed if desired and must be removed if a positive end-expiratory pressure (PEEP) valve is used because a PEEP valve goes on the expiratory port.

The PEEP valve itself is a disposable plastic device that looks similar to a heat and moisture exchanger filter. It has a spring-loaded disc inside it that resists expiratory flow, thereby causing PEEP. By twisting the PEEP valve, specific PEEP values can be "dialed in" along its indicator.

Function of the Bag Valve Mask

As mentioned, the internal volume of a self-inflating bag can be between 1500 and 2000 mL. Tidal volumes of this size cannot, however, be delivered by a BVM. In the best hands (pun intended), compressing the bag with both hands will not even deliver half of the resting volume of a BVM. One-handed bagging will deliver even less. A good compression will usually deliver anywhere from 500 to 800 mL.

The fraction of inspired oxygen (FiO_2) depends on two things: the rate of oxygen flow (liters per minute) from the flowmeter and the number of breaths per minute. Remember that when the bag inflates, it gets some volume from the gas tubing and some volume from the corrugated reservoir tubing. Smaller flows from the source cause the bag to entrain room air when it refills because there is not enough oxygen flow to fill it. This is remedied by using high flows (e.g., 10–15 L/min). The excess oxygen will fill the corrugated reservoir tubing, and the bag will entrain more oxygen than room air when it refills.

Similarly, rapid ventilation (e.g., 15–20 breaths/min) will decrease FiO_2 delivered to the patient. Naturally, if the patient needs to be hyperventilated, then you should hyperventilate. But what happens often is that from excitement during an acute situation or just not paying attention while transporting, we squeeze the bag too rapidly. This rapid rate depletes the corrugated reservoir tubing of its oxygen by not allowing enough time for it to fill with oxygen between breaths. As a result, room air is entrained when the bag inflates.

On some anesthesia machines, specifically those with a common gas outlet, inhalational agents can be delivered by a BVM. The BVM tubing will attach to a pediatric-sized ET tube adapter, which will fit perfectly into the common gas outlet. There should, however, be some means to scavenge the waste gas.

It is possible for the patient to spontaneously breathe when attached to a BVM. The dead space of the device is between 5 and 10 mL. What can happen, however, is failure of the nonrebreathing valve. The fishmouth-flap valve was designed for delivering positive-pressure ventilation to the patient. When the patient generates negative inspiratory force, the disc flap portion of the valve may become incompetent, leading to inspiration of room air through the expiratory port, causing a decrease in inspired oxygen content.

Hazards of the Bag Valve Mask

As with all medical devices, harm can happen during use. The BVM is no exception. Barotrauma can occur with the use of a BVM. Nonrebreathing valves can malfunction because of manufacturing problems, moisture, secretion, and so on. It is easy to forget to turn on the oxygen tank during transport. "Vigilance" is the one-word motto of the American Board of Anesthesiology for a reason. Whatever can go wrong will go wrong at some time.

It is our hope that you know much more now about how a BVM works. The next time you use one, you will perhaps have a greater appreciation of it and how such a simple device plays such a large role in our ability to care for seriously ill patients.

MAPLESON CIRCUITS

The Mapleson classification of circuits is something that has historically been very confusing to those learning anesthesia. Many of them are of historic interest only by now, and it has been difficult to remember the specifics about the different circuits.

There were various circuits already in clinical use when an anesthesiologist named William Mapleson at the University of Cardiff in Wales decided to classify them by position of the fresh gas flow (FGF) and the exhaust (or adjustable pressure-limiting [APL] valve) in an effort to determine how to decrease rebreathing. Keep in mind this was before the circle circuit was in common use. In his original classification, there were five classes, Mapleson A through E. The only circuits from the Mapleson classification that you are likely to see are the Jackson Rees (Mapleson F), the Bain circuit (Mapleson D variant), and the Mapleson E "T" piece.

Table 19-2 shows all Mapleson circuits and the minimum FGF needed for not rebreathing in spontaneous or controlled (manual) ventilation.

Mapleson F Circuit (Jackson Rees)

The Jackson Rees circuit is part of the *Mapleson classification*, specifically a modification of the Mapleson E circuit. A Mapleson E circuit is a simple T piece, and the modification is the addition of a reservoir bag to the distal limb of the T piece. The Jackson Rees circuit is so much different from the

Table 19-2 CLASSIFICATION AND CHARACTERISTICS OF MAPLESON CIRCUITS

Mapleson Class	Other Names	Configuration	Required Fresh Gas Flows		Comments
			Spontaneous	Controlled	
A	Magill attachment		Equal to minute ventilation (≈80 mL/kg/min)	Very high and difficult to predict	Poor choice during controlled ventilation. Enclosed Magill system is a modification that improves efficiency. Coaxial Mapleson A (Lack breathing system) provides waste-gas scavenging.
B			2 × minute ventilation	2–2½ × minute ventilation	
C	Waters' to-and-fro		2 × minute ventilation	2–2½ × minute ventilation	

D		2–3 × minute ventilation	1–2 × minute ventilation	Bain coaxial modification: fresh gas tube inside breathing tube
E	Ayre's T piece	2–3 × minute ventilation	3 × minute ventilation (I:E = 1:2)	Exhalation tubing should provide a larger volume than tidal volume to prevent rebreathing. Scavenging is difficult.
F	Jackson-Rees' modification	2–3 × minute ventilation	2 × minute ventilation	A Mapleson E with a breathing bag connected to the end of the breathing tube to allow controlled ventilation and scavenging

APL, adjustable pressure-limiting; FGI, fresh gas inlet.
Reproduced with permission from Morgan GE, Mikhail MS, Murray MI. *Clinical Anesthesiology.* 2nd ed. New York, NY: McGraw-Hill; 2002. Table 3-2.

Mapleson E, however, that it is given its own classification as a Mapleson F circuit. More or less, it is a T piece that has a manual bag on the end of the distal section of the T. There is a small release valve on the distal end of the bag itself that is used as a "pop off," enabling the user to roughly control volume and pressure of each bag compression. The reason that pediatric anesthesiologists often prefer this over a neonatal-sized BVM is that a Jackson Rees circuit gives you more "feel" of lung stiffness or compliance with each squeeze than a BVM does. This is similar to the difference in how ventilation feels when you ventilate an adult patient with your anesthesia circuit instead of a BVM. The stiffness of the BVM does not give an experienced hand the same tactile input that the circle circuit does.

Mapleson D Circuit (Bain)

We mentioned that another Mapleson class circuit that is still in use is a Bain circuit. So what exactly is a Bain circuit? It is a modification of a Mapleson D circuit. So what does *that* mean? A Mapleson D circuit is shown in Figure 19-5.

Notice that the fresh gas inlet for FGF is next to the patient end of the circuit (illustrated by a mask; it could be a laryngeal mask airway [LMA] or an ET tube for that matter). The APL, or "pop-off," valve is at the proximal end close to the reservoir bag. Because the FGF is close to the patient, it actually helps *blow away* the expired gas from the patient and toward the APL valve. This helps decrease the amount of rebreathing. Other Mapleson circuits have the FGF inlet farther away from the patient end.

A Bain circuit is a Mapleson D circuit that has the FGF tubing *inside* the expiratory limb, forming a *coaxial circuit*. Because of their compactness, Bain circuits are good to use when you do not have a regular anesthesia machine or you are in a place where a regular anesthesia machine will not fit. The circuit is mounted on a special yoke that has an adaptor for the reservoir bag, an APL valve, and an airway pressure gauge. The yoke can be attached to an intravenous pole or supply cart. Oxygen tubing from a wall or cylinder flowmeter attaches to the FGF inlet. It is possible to modify a Bain to deliver inhalational agents and to scavenge waste anesthetic agents.

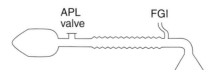

Figure 19-5 ■ Mapleson D circuit. Note that the fresh gas inlet (FGI) is distal to the adjustable pressure-limiting (APL) valve and proximal to the patient end. (Reproduced with permission from Morgan GE, Mikhail MS, Murray MJ. *Clinical Anesthesiology.* 2nd ed. New York, NY: McGraw-Hill; 2002. Table 3-2.)

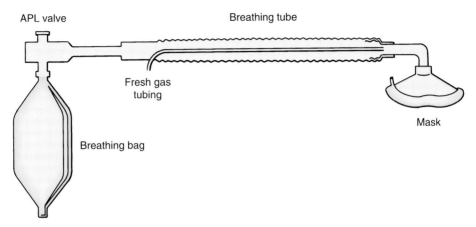

Figure 19-6 ■ A Bain circuit is a Mapleson D circuit design with the fresh gas tubing inside the corrugated breathing tube. APL, adjustable pressure-limiting. (Reproduced with permission from Morgan GE, Mikhail MS, Murray MJ. *Clinical Anesthesiology.* 2nd ed. New York, NY: McGraw-Hill; 2002. Figure 3-7.)

To decrease rebreathing, large FGFs are needed. You cannot use low flows like with a circle anesthesia circuit because the only way to avoid rebreathing is to have a FGF above minute ventilation. If a patient is spontaneously breathing with a Bain, the FGF needs to be two to three times the minute ventilation. For manual ventilation, the flow needs to be between one and two times the FGF. Some people may mistakenly think the coaxial circuit, with the fresh gas (or inspiratory) limb surrounded by the expiratory limb, may help in warming the inspired gas. But that is not true because of the high FGFs needed in a Bain circuit.

A schematic of a Bain circuit is shown in Figure 19-6.

Mapleson E Circuit (T Piece)

The third Mapleson circuit you will still see is the simple T piece. It is a Mapleson E circuit. In the table of Mapleson circuits, the Mapleson E doesn't look like just a T piece, but functionally, that is what it is. Of course, we think of using a T piece on a patient who is still intubated or even has an LMA in place instead of being used with a facemask. In addition, there is no reservoir bag to use for manual ventilation. It is simply a system to deliver oxygen right to the tip of the ET tube or LMA. The reservoir tubing on the other side of the T is there simply to act as a reservoir for oxygen, similar to the corrugated tubing we talked about earlier that you see on BVMs (Figure 19-7).

If the reservoir tubing was not there, with each spontaneous inspiration, the patient would be getting some of the inspired volume from the T end where the oxygen tubing is and some from entraining a great deal of room air.

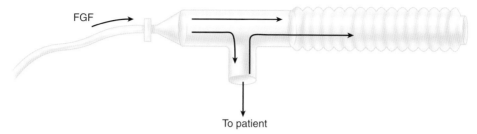

FGF

To patient

Figure 19-7 ▪ Diagram of a T piece (Mapleson E circuit). Note the corrugated tubing at the distal end of circuit, which acts as an oxygen reservoir and keeps room air from being entrained. FGF, fresh gas flow.

So after expiration, the distal tubing is full of carbon dioxide. But it fills quickly with oxygen from the FGF, so on the next inspiration, the extra tubing distal to the T contains a large amount of oxygen, so the FiO_2 is greatly increased. The longer the distal tubing, the greater the FiO_2 will be. But of course, the FGF needs to be of sufficient volume to flush the carbon dioxide from the distal tubing, or rebreathing will occur.

As mentioned, there is no reservoir bag on a T piece, but that does not mean there is no way to ventilate using positive-pressure ventilation. By closing off the expiratory limb with your hand, you will be able to ventilate a patient. We do not recommend this because there is no way to accurately measure the tidal volume given or to measure the airway pressure generated. Levels of airway pressure could be reached that would cause barotrauma. But in a true emergency with no other option, it is possible until a better means of positive-pressure ventilation is present, such as a BVM or a ventilator.

CONCLUSION

Now you should know how the three commonly used Mapleson circuits work. You may have even used them in the past without knowing that indeed they were Mapleson circuits. We hope we have decreased some of the difficulty in understanding this classification system for you by showing you real-life examples of their use.

SUGGESTED READING

1. Dorsch JA, Dorsch SE. Understanding Anesthesia Equipment. 5th Edition. 2007, Lippincott Williams & Wilkins.

WARMING DEVICES AND TEMPERATURE MONITORING

20

KEYWORDS

- temperature monitoring
- heat loss mechanisms
- warming devices
- types of warming devices
- efficacy of warming devices
- complications of warming devices
- blood warmers

Perioperative patient temperature changes are a "hot" topic now. Numerous studies over the past decade have shown a relationship between patient hypothermia and surgical wound infection and length of hospital stay in addition to the things related to patient temperature that have been long known, such as shivering, cardiovascular stress, coagulopathies, and patient satisfaction. The importance of regulation of room temperature for patient normothermia instead of staff comfort has been recognized. Some medical insurance companies audit perioperative patient temperature as an indicator of appropriate care for reimbursement.

Several methods are used to keep patients normothermic in the perioperative period. Some work much better than others. Some provide active warming, but some are passive in nature. We will talk about the different kinds of patient heat loss, as well as the different methods and the efficacy of each.

METHODS OF PERIOPERATIVE HEAT LOSS

Intuitively, it is not hard to understand why patients get cold perioperatively. You are placed in a cold room, told to take off your clothes, and put on a flimsy short-sleeve gown that is open in the back. You may or may not have a blanket.

Then you are given intravenous (IV) fluid that is room temperature. You are wheeled down a cold, drafty hallway into a cold room and placed on a cold bed. You are given drugs that negatively alter your body's thermoregulation. Then after you are unconscious, you are uncovered totally, positioned, washed in room temperature solution, and given more room temperature IV fluid. By the time you are covered up in surgical drapes, your temperature has dropped at least 1°C. The length and location of the operation will affect the degree of hypothermia, as well as the amount of IV fluid. You will lose 0.25°C of body temperature for every liter of room temperature IV fluid given. So it is easily understood why you get cold. But what are the methods of heat loss, speaking in terms of physics?

The four main methods of heat loss in an anesthetized patient are *radiation, conduction, convection*, and *evaporation*. You may not remember the differences in these, so we will go over each one.

Radiation

For this form of heat loss, think of heat as light (they both are energy, of course). In this example, the patient emits heat by radiation just like a light bulb emits light into the room. The colder the environment, the more heat is radiated away from the patient. This is actually the main way a patient loses heat.

Conduction

This is when heat energy flows from one molecule to another or one object to another. Contact is needed for heat loss to occur by conduction. The heat energy flows from the warmer to the colder object. The best example for us in the operating room (OR) is when the patient loses heat to the cold IV fluid that was just infused into him or her. The colder IV fluid molecules are in contact with warmer molecules that make up the patient, so heat is lost to the cold IV fluid, resulting in a decrease in overall temperature. Of course, the drop depends on how cold the IV fluid was and how much fluid is given.

Convection

In convection, heat is lost to moving air; it is the OR equivalent of the wind-chill factor. The amount of loss depends on the amount of draft and the temperature of the air.

Evaporation

In Chapter 6 on vaporizers, we mentioned that evaporation of our liquid anesthetic agent takes energy and that energy comes from the ambient temperature of the room where our vaporizer is. The heat of the room is used to cause vaporization of the agent.

The best example of evaporative heat loss is sweating. Why do we sweat when we are hot? It is a way to cool the body by evaporation. It takes energy to vaporize the liquid perspiration on our skin, and that energy comes from the heat of our body. Although our patients might not sweat, they nevertheless do have some heat loss occur through vaporization. The loss is more pronounced if the patient or drapes are wet, with the wetness acting similar to perspiration.

METHODS OF PATIENT WARMING

It does not take a professor of thermodynamics to tell us what we can do to keep a patient's heat loss to a minimum. Much of it is common sense. The patient should be kept as warm as possible preoperatively, in the holding room, and on the way to the OR. The OR should be as warm as possible while the patient is being anesthetized, positioned, and prepped. The patient should be covered as much as possible during induction, positioning, and prepping. Only after the patient is fully draped should lowering the room temperature be considered.

You can divide methods of warming two ways; there are *active* and *passive* methods, or you can think about warming the patient and warming IV fluids as two separate ways. Active methods include forced-air warmers, IV fluid warmers, and the like; passive methods include blankets and other coverings. Passive methods rely on trapping the heat being lost by the patient in the small envelope of air under the coverings.

Forced-Air Warmers

Often generically called "Bair huggers," after a certain brand, forced-air warmers are a very effective way to either warm a patient or keep a patient warm. A specially designed disposable plastic and paper drape is placed on the patient and attached to the unit that blows warmed air into the drape, dispersing the warm air to all parts of the drape. The air used is sucked into the unit, passing through a bacterial filter, warmed using a heater (with different temperature settings) in the unit, and taken to the drape via a hose. The drapes come in different sizes and shapes to allow for differences in patient size and operative area. Some drapes are designed to go under the patient, around the patient, or over the patient. There are even robe-like drapes that can be used in the holding room to decrease heat loss preoperatively.

There are several advantages to forced-air warmers. As mentioned, they are a very effective means of temperature control in the OR, better than other types in many studies. After the unit has been bought, the cost of using a forced-air warmer is low. The drapes, although only for one-time use, are relatively inexpensive and can be charged to the patient and can go from holding to the OR to recovery with the patient if desired. The units are thermostatically controlled to keep the unit and air from getting too hot. An "ambient" setting on many units will blow room temperature air through the drape if a patient gets too warm during a procedure. Some are designed to allow IV tubing to be warmed also. Using a forced-air warmer can allow the room temperature to be lowered, making gowned personnel more comfortable.

The disadvantages of forced-air warmers themselves are few if they are used properly. The main problem is the risk of patient burns if the warmer is used incorrectly. A forced-air warmer should never be used on a patient without the special warmer drape. As mentioned, the drape disperses the heat evenly so there are no "hot points," areas where more of the warmer output lands and causes burns. There are case reports of the warmer being used by putting the output hose between the patient's legs and covering the patient with a blanket (hosing). This concentrates the warmed air, and burns can occur; even though the maximum temperature setting is 43°C, the air coming out of the hose is 3° to 5°C warmer than the set temperature, and it cools as it is dispersed by the special blanket. Other problems can occur from using a unit and hose from different manufacturers (comingling). There is even a website to educate users about the dangers of hosing, called stophosing.com.

In addition to burns from hosing, the hose itself can get warm enough to burn a patient if left on the same site for an extended time. Extremities below a vascular clamp can be burned because there is no blood flow to circulate the warmth. Forced-air warmers add to the noise of an OR (but the benefit to the patient greatly outweighs the noise pollution problem). Forced-air warmers are not magnetic resonance imaging compatible; the blanket is, but the unit is not.

Water Blanket Warmers

These units were used commonly before the advent of forced-air warmers. A specially designed watertight pad is placed under the bedsheets of the OR table. This pad is attached to a warming unit by two tubes, and warm water is circulated through the pad and back to the warming unit. In addition to warming, the unit could be used to cool the patient. These devices are less effective than forced-air warmers.

Conductive Fabric Blankets

This is a relatively new method of patient warming. A special conductive fabric blanket has electricity sent through it. The large electrical resistance of the fabric generates heat. Sensors control how much electricity is sent through the fabric in order to maintain a safe, steady temperature.

These blankets are reusable. The system is ungrounded, so there is no danger of electrical shock to the patient or personnel. One example of a conductive blanket system is called "Hot Dog." The manufacturer claims there is less incidence of orthopedic wound infection with their device than a standard forced-air warmer because the forced-air warmer creates convection air currents that can spread fomites up into the surgical site.

Radiant Heating Lights

"French fry lights" are often used in pediatric cases. They can be used for adults as well, but the large surface area of infants means the radiant lights are more effective than for adults. The best results are obtained when the patient is uncovered totally. The lights are on a panel or an IV pole, with a measuring stick attached, because if the lights are in too close proximity to the patient burns can occur. Care must be taken because the lights can melt plastic IV bags or burst glass IV bottles or even burn personnel if the bulbs are touched. They are less effective than forced-air warmers.

Heated Anesthesia Circuits

These units were common in ORs 20 years ago but are less common now. They will be seen more frequently in critical care settings. A heated humidifier is attached to the inspiratory limb of the circle circuit, and as the inspiratory flow flows over the heated water, both heating and humidification occur. A temperature feedback probe is placed at the Y piece to regulate the temperature.

Heated humidifiers had many drawbacks for use in anesthesia. One thing was that they were not very effective. Again, forced-air warming is far superior. Second, use of a heated humidifier multiplied the places for and chances of a circuit disconnect. There were more places to become disconnected, and the warmth and moisture of the circuit adapters made a disconnect occur more easily. Third, if a heated humidifier was improperly attached, the circuit could melt, causing a catastrophic loss of positive pressure in the circuit. One of the authors witnessed a STAT call to an OR, where the circuit had been melted apart because the provider had not placed the temperature sensor in the Y piece, so the heater kept on getting warmer and warmer, with no feedback from the sensor, until the plastic circuit melted. You should be glad these devices are no longer in common use.

Heat and Moisture Exchanger

A heat and moisture exchanger (HME) is a small, filter-like attachment to the anesthesia circuit that is supposed to fit between the endotracheal tube or supraglottic device and the Y piece. Its 15-mm fittings allow it to be placed only in that area. It is similar to the filters discussed in the Chapter 7 on the anesthesia circuit and is made of either hydrophobic or hygroscopic material to catch exhaled moisture and allow it to be delivered back to the patient with subsequent inspirations. A common design of hydrophobic HME will contain what looks like a roll of corrugated paper inside it to trap the exhaled moisture. But because it is hydrophobic, the water that is trapped is not absorbed into the paper but stays on the outside of the paper.

Heat and moisture exchangers are designed to have low resistance to breathing. There are different sizes available for adult and pediatric patients. An HME that is too small will be inefficient, but one that is too large (e.g., an adult-sized HME for a child) will increase dead space.

Perhaps they should be called "MEs" because the ability of them to conserve H (heat) is limited. You will not warm up a cold patient by placing an HME. But they do a good job in increasing the moisture content of the inhaled gas between the HME and the patient's lungs in cases longer than a few minutes.

The HME should be placed distal to any sidestream gas monitoring sample line take off because if the gas sample is taken from the area between the HME and the patient, excess water can be drawn off, interfering with the gas monitor or requiring you to empty or replace the gas monitor water trap frequently. Excess water, sputum, blood, or any other fluid in the circuit can increase resistance and even cause obstruction and increase peak airway pressures.

Blankets

Blankets are low tech, safe, and require no training to use. Although they are better than nothing, they do have limited value. This type of passive heating relies on insulation, trapping the thin layer of warm air next to the patient and keeping it there. Heated blankets may be psychologically appealing, but their efficacy is no better than unheated blankets after the first few minutes. Additional layers of covering are minimally better than a single layer. Blankets are no better than surgical drapes or reflective "space" or "survival" type blankets in the OR setting.

Low Fresh Gas Flow and Coaxial Circuits

As discussed in other chapters, these two modalities may decrease the amount of temperature drop but will not warm a patient.

Warm Intravenous Bags

In this case, we mean using warm IV bags *externally* like you would use an old-fashioned hot water bottle. We mention this as a warning: *do not* do this!

It may seem like a great idea to heat IV bags in a microwave oven or keep some in a blanket warmer cabinet and then use the warm bags to nestle next to a patient or to use a warm IV bag as an axillary roll for a laterally positioned patient. This is a very easy way to cause burns to the patient.

METHODS OF INTRAVENOUS FLUID WARMING

Warm IV fluid will not warm up a patient who is hypothermic unless large amounts of fluid are being infused. Its main role is to prevent further loss of body temperature from fluid that is room temperature, or in the case of blood products, frankly cold. That being said, we certainly advocate the use of fluid warmers when infusing large amounts of IV fluid or any time cold blood products are given. But their use otherwise is not clear-cut, and many clinicians do not use fluid warming devices for cases not requiring volume resuscitation or transfusion.

There are a few things that influence the effectiveness of IV fluid warmers. One thing is the initial temperature of the fluid. In most cases except for blood, the fluid will be room temperature. Another factor is the flow rate. If you are only infusing 500 mL over an hour to an adult patient, the fluid will probably return to close to room temperature by the time it reaches the patient after leaving the warmer. Yet another factor is the length of the IV tubing from the warmer to the patient. Longer tubing means the fluid will lose more heat as it is being infused regardless of the flow rate. The final thing to consider is the temperature that the warmer is set for.

There are multiple means of warming fluid and blood for IV use. Crystalloid can be kept in blanket-warming cabinets and infused. The patient will not get warmer, but it will decrease the rate of temperature loss. Much of the warmth of the fluid is lost along the tubing from the bag to the patient. Using a microwave oven to warm IV fluid bags has been done, but the fluid can get too warm. There are also cases of people microwaving units of blood, causing erythrocyte lysis and hyperkalemia.

The safest way to warm fluid for IV use is with a dedicated fluid warming system. Several different technologies are used in fluid warmers for ORs, emergency departments, and critical care units. Commonly, the devices are set to deliver IV fluid that is 41°C when the fluid leaves the unit.

Dry Heat Plates

In this method, a flat "cassette" of the same material that IV tubing is made from is placed between two flat plates that are heated. The flow rate is less than on other types, but nevertheless, this is an effective means of warming

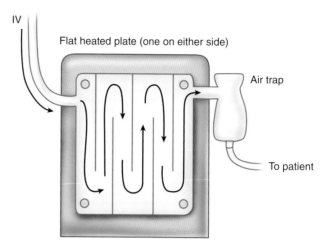

Figure 20-1 ▪ Dry heat fluid warmer. The front side is not shown for clarity. The cassette fits between the two warming plates like a piece of paper between the halves of a book. IV, intravenous.

IV fluid. Care must be taken, as in all IV tubing, to prime the cassette to rid it of all air (Figure 20-1).

Countercurrent Warmers

This type of warmer is similar to a coaxial anesthesia circle circuit, with one tube inside of another. In this case, the tubing inside is the path of the IV fluid. The outer tubing or jacket contains circulating warm distilled water that heats the IV fluid as the IV fluid flows through the inner tubing. Generally, these types of warmers allow more rapid infusion rates than the dry heat plate types. Some are marketed for use in trauma resuscitation (level one warmers), with the ability to pressurize the IV bags through the medical air pipeline outlet. There is also some form of air trap or air detector to prevent inadvertent air embolism from rapid infusion. Regardless, bags of fluid or blood products should be vented to remove all air in them when any form of pressurization of IV lines is done. Detectors and air traps can be overwhelmed or malfunction, and even a vigilant clinician can overlook air in the line, especially when busy during volume resuscitation (Figure 20-2).

Microwave Warmers

We discussed the use of a microwave oven for warming fluid, but in this instance, we mean a dedicated inline specifically designed unit that uses microwaves to

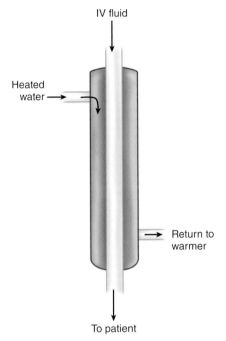

IV fluid

Heated
water →

Return to
warmer

To patient

Figure 20-2 ■ Countercurrent fluid warmer. The outer jacket of warm distilled water heats the inner tubing containing intravenous fluid.

warm fluid. Sensors detect the temperature of the incoming fluid, the flow rate, and the temperature of the outgoing fluid and adjust the energy input of the microwave unit to keep the outgoing fluid at the set temperature.

TEMPERATURE MONITORING

Temperature monitoring is not needed in every anesthetic; for instance, it is not needed in a 20-minute cataract procedure on an adult done under monitored anesthesia care (MAC). But the *ability* to measure temperature for every case is a standard of care.

Most of the time, a type of special temperature probe with a thermistor that attaches to a monitor is used in anesthesia settings, but one could use any patient thermometer if needed. There are adhesive skin temperature probes also; they may be appropriate for MAC cases, but they can be difficult to read and may not reflect true core or blood temperature. Pulmonary artery catheters have a built-in thermistor. Bladder (Foley) catheters are available with incorporated temp probes. These are very useful in head and neck cases when there is no access to the patient's upper body.

For many years, temperature probes have been combined with esophageal stethoscopes. But because there has been a gradual decrease in the number of clinicians who listen to the patient throughout a procedure, many younger practitioners have no idea that the esophageal temperature probe is actually a stethoscope also. The authors enjoy asking a new resident why the esophageal temperature probe has an open end; the resident is then amazed when shown how to listen to the patient's lungs during the anesthetic. Even the package the combination stethoscope temperature probe will say something like "esophageal stethoscope with temperature probe," but people don't always read the package.

There are many places to measure temperature during an anesthetic. We have mentioned the esophagus, skin, blood, and bladder. Other sites include rectum, nasopharynx, and axilla. The standard adult-sized or pediatric esophageal stethoscope and temperature probe can be used, and some specialized probes for different sites are available as well, such as the ear canal (tympanic).

Hazards of temperature probes include the chance of causing bleeding, rare instances of burns, tissue trauma (lacerations, perforations), and false information. The authors have seen instances of falsely high and falsely low temperatures generated by disposable temperature probes. Another hazard, specifically in head and neck surgery, that we are aware of is surgical transection of a temperature probe.

CONCLUSION

We hope you put this information to use in your clinical practice. The importance of normothermia in surgical patients has finally been recognized. You now know the physics behind patient temperature loss, different methods of warming, and the hazards that can be encountered as well.

ELECTRICITY AND ELECTRICAL SAFETY IN THE OPERATING ROOM

21

As we all know, electrical equipment is a big part of our lives. At home, out and about, in hospitals and the operating room (OR), electricity is flowing and powering our lives. The OR is a special area with special electrical requirements and unique dangers that we will explore. Naturally, part of that discussion involves some basic physics about electricity and discussion about circuitry. Even as we go through the definitions, keep in mind why the discussion about electricity is important. Besides the fact that electricity powers most of the equipment in an OR, electricity can be a major source of injury to patients, staff, and us by fire or by shock (Figure 21-1).

BASICS

Let's start off with a classic equation of electricity, Ohm's law, which is $V = I \times R$. V is the force or voltage difference in volts, I is the current in amperes, and R is the resistance in ohms. If we rearrange the symbols to $I = E/R$, the flow, or current in amperes, is equal to the voltage difference divided by the resistance. So, the higher the voltage difference for a given resistance, the higher the flow of current is and vice versa. Following along in the equation, the higher the resistance for a given voltage, the lower the flow will be, and again, the

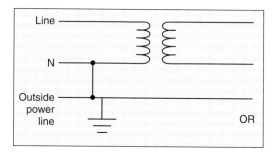

Figure 21-1 ▪ One-circuit configuration for operating room (OR) isolation.

reverse is also true. Another way to think of is to compare this to water behind a dam. As long as the dam is intact, there is no flow across the dam, but the water pressure behind the dam is still there. And the more water the dam is holding back, the higher the water pressure is behind the dam, and the more potential flow there would be if the dam were to fail. That is like the voltage in an electrical circuit. If there is a hole in the dam, then there will be flow, and that is similar to the amperage in the circuit (electrical current is electrons in motion). If you make a hole in a dam that has very little water behind it, the flow through the hole in the dam won't be as great compared with a dam that has a lot of water behind it. This is the same as in an electrical circuit, where the higher the voltage or potential difference is, the more current will flow for a given resistance. This example also holds up for resistance. If you make a huge hole in a dam, the resistance to water flow through the dam will be less than if the hole is really small so there would be more flow through the dam with the big hole. It's the same for electricity. The lower the resistance, the more flow there is for a given voltage.

There are only a few more terms we need to have clear in our minds. Wattage is electrical power, and its formula is $P = V \times I$. Because V is $I \times R$, wattage $= I^2 \times R$. The amount of work done by the electrical power is coupled with time. So a watt-second is called 1 joule. For the outside electrical wires that bring electricity to your house, the expression is in kilowatt-hours to accommodate higher amounts of energy. Impedance is applicable to AC circuits and is what opposes the flow of current in an AC circuit. Insulators have a high impedance, and conductors have a low impedance. Capacitance is the ability to store charge within a circuit. In all equipment, there is at least some stray capacitance, which means the equipment is able to hold a charge because it is made of conductors and insulators, not just because capacitors were built into its circuitry. Stray capacitance in electrical devices in the OR could cause a problem for OR personnel and especially patients with cardiac devices such as defibrillators. More on stray capacitance later.

So now we need to spend a little time talking about circuits. In its simplest form, an electrical circuit is a loop formed by wire that has a voltage source attached to it, like a battery. There is no flow of electricity if there is not a complete circuit leading to and from the voltage source. There is at least one other thing added to the circuit, and that something is what the electricity is powering, such as a light bulb, computer, or electrical appliance. The battery provides the voltage difference so that there is flow of electrons through the circuit, going to the appliance and returning to the battery. The higher the voltage is in the battery, the higher the flow will be for a given resistance (like the water behind the dam example we used earlier). Just a quick note about AC and DC circuits. There is a rich history in the United States of alternating current (AC) versus direct (DC) transmission on larger scales with AC eventually winning for reasons that aren't important for this discussion. What is important is that AC current is usually how electricity travels over wires in the United States, and AC current is also what is on both sides of the isolation transformer from the OR side. What is important about DC circuits is that is what is usually inside many of the everyday devices we use such as computers.

Let's talk a little bit about electrical ground or grounding. We have all heard about grounding, and it is important for us to have a basic understanding. If you think back to our discussion of a circuit, recall that a circuit is really just a loop for electrons or current to flow through. So there is a hot wire that brings the electricity to something and a neutral wire to bring the current back to its source, thus completing our loop or circuit. If the hot wire gets disrupted, there is no flow unless the current somehow finds a connection to the neutral wire or ground. But what happens if the neutral wire gets disrupted for some reason? Then the hot wire could bring the current to an appliance, casing, or outlet and charge it, and when you touch it, you could get shocked. There is a third wire, the grounding wire, that would take that stray current and send it to the earth ground, where it won't hurt anybody. In this way, if the neutral wire is disrupted, the current has somewhere to go because current is lazy and will follow the path of least resistance, and the ground wire is a very low-resistance place for it to go. So grounding helps prevent charge from getting stored up on appliances or other things. We will talk about implications for grounding in the OR in just a little bit.

RISK OF SHOCK

Before we head to the OR, let's spend a little time on electrical shock. So how do our patients, and we, get shocked? First of all, shock is electrical current applied to the body. How relevant that shock is to the patient or to us is dependent on several variables. First, where is the exposure? If it is to the

Table 21-1	MACROSHOCK ASSUMING 60-HZ ALTERNATING CURRENT
Milliamperes	**Effect**
1	Threshold of perception
5	Roughly the maximum harmless current intensity
~10–20	"Let-go" value; involuntary painful muscle contraction
~50	Pain; mechanical injury
~100	Ventricular fibrillation but respiratory center is intact
>6000	Sustained myocardial contraction; respiratory paralysis; burns if current density is high
Microshock	
Microamperes	**Effect**
~50–100	Ventricular fibrillation
10	Maximum allowable leakage current if in contact with the heart
2000	LIM warning level (no help against microshock)

LIM, line isolation monitor.

skin, it is called macroshock, and if it goes straight to the heart, it is called a microshock. Microshock could occur if there was an exposed pacemaker lead, for example. As you can imagine, it usually takes a lot more electricity to hurt someone in a macroshock situation than it does in a microshock situation. For instance, the human threshold for perception of electric current on dry skin is about 1 milliamp, which, applied to skin, is noticeable but not dangerous. If that current were applied to a wire connected directly to the heart, there is a very high chance it would cause ventricular fibrillation (Table 21-1).

The injury from an electric shock is also related to the current, or amperage, of the exposure, and as you would expect, the higher the current, the more dangerous the exposure. In addition, as you would expect, the longer the duration of exposure to electricity, the more damage there will be to tissues and to increase the chance of having dangerous or lethal arrhythmias.

A good example of macroshock from outside the OR is a lightning strike. People can get hurt if there is a direct strike or if a person is in contact with something that gets hit by lightning. We can even get hurt if we are standing close to a spot where lightning hits the ground. Lightning can kill us because it is typically a huge voltage that we get exposed to even though the exposure is brief. It can disrupt the conducting system of the heart and lead to a lethal arrhythmia. It can also cause life-threatening tissue damage to organs such as the heart, brain, aorta, or muscles by burning them. Short of death, lightning, as with any macro-shock, can also cause tissue damage that is permanent, especially to nerves and muscles because they are part of the body's electrical system.

OPERATING ROOM ELECTRICAL DESIGN

We've come a long way on our path to understanding some basics about electricity, so how are the circuits set up in the OR, and why did the engineers design it this way? Let's answer the second question first. The circuits are set up to make it very difficult for anyone in the OR to get shocked whether it is a patient, us, or other OR personnel. In addition, the engineers want to make it difficult for there to be a fire in the OR caused by an electrical issue.

Thinking back to our knowledge of Ohm's law and our knowledge of circuitry, a person can't get shocked unless he or she touches something that completes a circuit. Knowing this, the engineers set up the circuits in the OR to make it difficult for a person in the OR to complete a circuit and thus receive a shock. How did they do it? Well, it can be set up in different ways, but here is one. As the electrical current enters the hospital, the neutral and ground wires are electrically connected. As the electricity gets to the ORs, it hits an isolation transformer where the neutral line becomes ungrounded while the ground obviously stays grounded. So the circuits to the individual pieces of equipment in the OR are electrically isolated from the ground, which means it is much harder to get shocked. For someone to get shocked, he or she would have to be in contact with both the isolated circuit and the ground, which is hard to do but, of course, possible. This could happen if the insulation around the wires (hot, neutral, or ground) is not good. Another way would be if the wires in the OR or the ground wires were exposed in water and someone was in contact with the water. Because the circuits in the OR are ungrounded, what happens if, for instance, a metal casing around a piece of surgical equipment began to get charged because of a bad neutral wire? If we were at our house, the ground wire would take that charge to the ground and short out the circuit. In the OR, that is where the line isolation monitor comes into play. What is a line isolation monitor (LIM)? The LIM is placed to measure to see if the current going into a circuit is the same as it is going out and is typically set to detect very low amperage differences. It essentially functions as a comparator that compares the amperage coming into the OR and the amperage going out. If there is a difference, the LIM alarm will sound. What does that mean to us and to our patients? It means we need to look for a source of the lost current like we talked about earlier. It does not tell us which device or wire is causing the leak and will not prevent an electrical shock by itself but warns of the possibility of electrocution. Again, it *will not* cut off the flow of electricity, but it tells you to look for a source of possible electrocution. A good place to start looking is the last thing that was plugged in before the LIM alarm went off.

While we're talking about comparators, we need to talk about another kind of comparator in electrical circuits, a ground fault circuit interrupter (GFCI). The GFCI is basically another comparator like the LIM that continually compares the amperage going through a circuit after the electrical current goes through the devices in the circuit. The difference is the GFCI *will* break the current flow in the circuit to limit the exposure of electricity to a person. The GFCI is very fast and will stop current flow in several thousandths of a second when it detects an amperage difference between the ingoing and outgoing current, limiting exposure to the electrical current. So that ends our tour of electricity and circuits.

CONCLUSION

As you have probably noticed, one of the themes of this book is that we all stand on the shoulders of our predecessors, and our understanding of electricity and how our ORs are wired continues that theme. Numerous engineers over many years have continued to refine how we power the equipment in ORs while trying to protect everyone in those same ORs, and we should all be grateful for their efforts.

NEW DEVELOPMENTS IN ANESTHESIA EQUIPMENT | 22

KEYWORDS

- xenon
- vaporizer types
- flowmeters
- closed-loop anesthesia
- costs of anesthesia care

Did you ever see the movie *2001, A Space Odyssey*? Besides being known for giving us Ric Flair's entrance music, it is also known as a visionary film. Made in 1968 in the midst of the *Apollo* Program's efforts to land on the moon, one of the signature scenes is aboard a commercial space plane traveling from Earth to a space station. You see, in 1968, it did not seem far-fetched that by the end of the century humankind would have such things—space ports and scientific bases on the moon and maybe even Mars.

Why do we mention this? Because it shows how difficult it is to predict the future. Unless we missed the news report, we are still waiting for a base on the moon or a human trip to Mars. In the 1960s, those things seemed like they would have been a certainty 40 or 50 years later. So in this chapter, we are not going to predict what is in the future, but we will discuss some of the things that are *already* in use (in the section The Future is Now) or things that have been tested in the area of anesthesia equipment (in the section Not Anytime Soon).

THE FUTURE IS NOW

We say the future is now because there are some things that are already in limited use but have not fully penetrated the anesthesia equipment market. As is often the case, it takes a while for some new things to catch on or to prove their worth. This is how it was for pulse oximetry and capnography a generation ago. The automated record is another example of something that is readily available for purchase and use but is not universally used by anesthesia practitioners.

Xenon

Xenon is supposed to be the next big thing in anesthesia. This noble gas has many properties of the ideal inhalational agent. It is already in use clinically in Russia and Germany. In this section, we will not discuss the pharmacology and physiologic concerns of xenon but will focus on issues involving its supply and delivery.

The big problem with xenon is its rarity and its expense. You may recall that xenon is found in our atmosphere but in a very small concentration (0.0000087%, or 1 part per 11.5 million). In fact, the amount of xenon being produced each year currently is only enough for less than half a million anesthetics. It takes a lot of energy to separate 1 L of xenon from the atmosphere.

At the time this book is being written, 1 L of xenon in the United States costs $10 to $12 or so. Even with a closed-circuit technique and rebreathing, a xenon anesthetic would be expensive. Administration would be computer controlled; you dial in what concentration you want, and the circuitry would inject amounts of the gas to reach and maintain that concentration based on whatever the inspired and expired xenon concentration was. Delivery systems are in use or in development to make xenon a viable, less expensive anesthetic, mainly by recapturing xenon instead of letting it go into a scavenger system.

Besides cost and the need for special equipment to administer and re-collect it, there are other problems associated with the use of xenon as an anesthetic. One problem with xenon is how to measure its concentration while administering it. It cannot be measured by infrared anesthetic gas monitoring. It can be measured by a mass spectrometer (as discussed in Chapter 16 on capnography) or by a method called thermal conductivity. Another problem is the human quality of not wanting to try something new. At least when newer halogenated inhalational agents were introduced in the past, these agents used familiar-looking vaporizers and could be used on existing anesthesia machines. It is our feeling that xenon will probably not become as routine of an anesthetic as sevoflurane, desflurane, and so on because of the cost. Many worry about the effect of inhalational agents and nitrous oxide on the environment and hope that xenon will be able to replace those anesthetics to a great extent. Because xenon is present in the atmosphere anyway and in fact comes from atmospheric air, there would be no pollution from the release of xenon into the atmosphere. It is yet to be seen if enough xenon can be produced each year, however, to substantially decrease the use of nitrous oxide and halogenated agents worldwide and if the energy that would be expended on xenon production would be worse for the environment than the release of our current anesthetic agents into the atmosphere.

Total Hemoglobin Monitoring

Total hemoglobin monitoring, or SpHb, is an exciting technology that has become available recently. In short, this monitor allows you to continuously monitor hemoglobin during a case. The technology is similar to that of pulse oximetry in which light of known wavelengths travel through a vascular bed (e.g. a finger), and a photodiode on the other side detects the light that made it through, giving you an approximate hemoglobin concentration. This is called *spectrophotometry*, and it is covered in more detail in Chapter 17 on pulse oximetry. There are different manufacturers of this technology, and the data suggest that the accuracy is not perfect but is acceptable to hemoglobin levels from a blood sample sent to the lab. It is safe to say that SpHb monitoring will be more commonly used in anesthetics when blood loss is a major concern.

Electronic Control of Vaporizers and Flowmeters

In earlier chapters, we talked about how anesthesia machines are becoming more and more dependent on electricity to work; some things that work fine without electric power now are being changed to require electricity to function. Vaporizers and flowmeters are perfect examples. Again, this is not something that will happen in the future. There are machines on the market right now that use this.

The most modern vaporizers are connected to sensors on the inspiratory and expiratory limbs of the circle circuit to more accurately deliver the concentration of agent that you have dialed in based on the fresh gas flow (FGF) that you are using. So that means that when you first turn on such a vaporizer, the output *may be more* than you have dialed in to more quickly obtain equilibrium with what concentration you actually want. Also, if you change the FGF, the vaporizer knows it and will correspondingly change its output to keep the agent concentration you have selected. A similar system now exists for flowmeters to more accurately and quickly change the concentration of gases whenever it is changed.

ANESTHESIA WORKSTATION

This is a phrase that simply means that the anesthetic machine and accompanying monitors are integrated into one unit. You can buy a machine and the monitors you need piecemeal, selecting the ones that you think are best or the best value for your group, or just get a new machine and keep the monitors you have now. *Or* you can purchase an anesthesia workstation with everything in one big unit. In workstations, there may be more *connectivity* between monitors (more on that later).

NOT ANYTIME SOON

Connectivity

"The operating room of the future" is a misnomer. It does not exist in the future; it exists now. What are we talking about?

At the Massachusetts General Hospital, a project called "The Operating Room of the Future" has been a test bed for new ideas for not only anesthesia technology but also surgery. One of the big concepts from this project is "plug and play." What this means is that *all* anesthesia equipment should be able to talk to each other.

Let's make up two anesthesia equipment companies, ACME and A-1. Now if you have an ACME anesthesia machine and an A-1 capnometer, there is no communication from one to another. Each unit has software and hardware that makes them incompatible. But what if you could tell the capnometer that you want the end-tidal carbon dioxide level to be maintained at 35 mm Hg? If the two units communicated, the capnometer could tell the anesthesia machine ventilator to increase or decrease minute ventilation to keep the end-tidal carbon dioxide where you want it. Of course, you would also program in parameters for the ventilator as well, such as not to exceed a certain peak airway pressure, and so forth. That is an example of "plug and play."

Here is another more practical example; you buy a new printer for your computer. You get it home and unpack it but only then do you realize that the printer is not compatible with your computer. Fortunately, this does not happen very often because of standardization with computer ports, such as USB. So *why* can't we make anesthesia equipment the same way?

The answer is that *we can*. There only needs to be industry standards for software and port compatibility. If the computer industry did it, the medical companies should be able to also. So in the near future, you will see "plug and play" becomes a more important concept in not only anesthesia equipment but all other medical equipment.

Closed-Loop Anesthesia

The technology exists, and has even been tested on humans, that allows a computer to control and adjust the infusion of anesthesia medications. Using total intravenous anesthesia (TIVA) with infusion pumps, systems have been able to titrate propofol, narcotic, and muscle relaxant infusions based on vital signs, electroencephalography (EEG), and nerve stimulator information. One such system is called "McSleepy." Closed-loop anesthesia could be easily adapted to use inhalational agents, especially with newer vaporizers that are electronically controlled. So does this mean we are all going to be replaced by robots?

Well, we think, not for a while. What may happen, ideally, is that the titration we do routinely now will be done automatically in the future under our supervision and under patient parameters prescribed and controlled by us. Then we would have more time to take care of the patient instead of having to perform the mundane task of anesthetic titration.

Of course, this concept not only opens up a can of worms, but it opens up a lot of cans of worms. A decrease in vigilance could be the true outcome. Is the titration of anesthesia really a mundane task, or is it part of what we are and how we learn what our drugs do? What happens if the intravenous line infiltrates? If we rely too much on automation, will we lose our clinical skills? As you see, this may be an example of technology developing more quickly than our ability to use it. But closed-loop anesthesia will play some role in our specialty in the future.

Teleanesthesia

Although it is technologically possible, or will soon be possible, for an anesthesiologist to intubate or even perform an epidural or nerve block remotely by robotic means, we must ask ourselves is this really necessary. What teleanesthesia's greatest boon may be is for real-time remote consultation.

Let's think of an example. You are anesthetizing someone in a small community hospital. She develops a dysrhythmia that you cannot figure out. Or you have a blood gas result that is perplexing. Or you want to start a pressor on a patient but are not sure which drug would be the best choice. Via instant messaging with an anesthesia faculty member at an academic institution with expertise in what you want to know, you discuss what to do remotely. The consultant on the other end has a screen with all the vital signs, capnography information, and laboratory values plus a camera to look at the patient. This is a good example of the "connectivity" that we discussed earlier.

Although there would be medicolegal problems to work through, it is not unreasonable to consider a "network" of community hospitals that contract with an academic or large group anesthesia practice to provide this remote consultation in the near future.

End-Tidal Propofol

When using a propofol infusion, we have no information on really how much is in a patient's system. We are "flying blind" somewhat similar to what practitioners did before end-tidal anesthetic agent monitoring was commonplace. Depth of anesthesia with propofol is determined by vital signs, EEG, and the presence or absence of movement, just like clinicians using inhalational agent a generation ago.

Propofol has enough of a volatile property that it can be detected in a patient's breath. Studies confirm that there is a relationship between end-tidal propofol concentration and plasma concentration. What is needed now is a reliable, efficient means of measuring propofol. Current infrared gas monitoring would be unable to measure the drug. The studies used mass spectrometry to obtain the information. If practical, end-tidal measurement of propofol for clinical purposes would be a generational achievement similar to the introduction of pulse oximetry and capnography.

| CONCLUSION

Compared with some specialties in medicine, new developments in anesthesia occur infrequently. But when they do happen, the developments have major implications. Don't forget how much has changed in the course of the time span of a career. There are still current practitioners out there who, at the start of their career, used ether. Even clinicians in the middle of their professional life have seen big changes. It will be interesting to see what will cause the next substantial change in our practice.

Index

Note: Page numbers followed by *f* denote figures; page numbers followed by *t* denote tables.